Conceptual Advances in Pathology

Editor

ZOLTÁN N. OLTVAI

CLINICS IN LABORATORY MEDICINE

www.labmed.theclinics.com

Consulting Editor
ALAN WELLS

December 2012 • Volume 32 • Number 4

ELSEVIER

1600 John F. Kennedy Boulevard • Suite 1800 • Philadelphia, Pennsylvania 19103-2899

http://www.theclinics.com

CLINICS IN LABORATORY MEDICINE Volume 32, Number 4
December 2012 ISSN 0272-2712, ISBN-13: 978-1-4557-4959-1

Editor: Teia Stone

Reprints. For copies of 100 or more, of articles in this publication, please contact the Commercial Reprints Department, Elsevier Inc., 360 Park Avenue South, New York, New York 10010-1710. Tel. (212) 633-3813, Fax: (212) 462-1935, E-mail: reprints@elsevier.com.

Clinics in Laboratory Medicine (ISSN 0272-2712) is published quarterly by Elsevier Inc., 360 Park Avenue South, New York, NY 10010-1710. Months of issue are March, June, September, and December. Business and Editorial offices: 1600 John F. Kennedy Blvd., Suite 1800, Philadelphia, PA 19103-2899. Periodicals postage paid at NewYork, NY and additional mailing offices. Subscription prices are $240.00 per year (US individuals), $382.00 per year(US institutions), $128.00(US students), $291.00 per year (Canadian individuals), $483.00 per year (foreign institutions), $176.00 (foreign students). Foreign air speed delivery is included in all Clinics subscription prices. All prices are subject to change without notice. POSTMASTER: Send address changes to *Clinics in Laboratory Medicine*, Elsevier Health Sciences Division, Subscription Customer Service, 3251 Riverport Lane, Maryland Heights, MO 63043. **Customer Service: 1-800-654-2452 (US). From outside of the US and Canada, call 1-314-447-8871. Fax: 1-314-447-8029. E-mail: journalscustomer service-usa@elsevier.com (for print support) or journalsonlinesupport-usa@elsevier.com (for online support).**

Clinics in Laboratory Medicine is covered in *EMBASE/Exerpta Medica*, *MEDLINE/PubMed (Index Medicus)*, *Cinahl*, *Current Contents/Clinical Medicine*, *BIOSIS* and *ISI/BIOMED*.

Printed and bound by CPI Group (UK) Ltd, Croydon, CR0 4YY

Transferred to digital print 2012

Contributors

CONSULTING EDITOR

ALAN WELLS, MD
Professor and Vice Chair, Department of Pathology, University of Pittsburgh Medical Center, Pittsburgh, Pennsylvania

GUEST EDITOR

ZOLTÁN N. OLTVAI, MD
Associate Professor, Department of Pathology, University of Pittsburgh Medical Center, Pittsburgh, Pennsylvania

AUTHORS

M.J. BECICH, MD, PhD
Department of Biomedical Informatics and Department of Pathology, University of Pittsburgh School of Medicine, University of Pittsburgh Cancer Institute, Pittsburgh, Pennsylvania

R. DHIR, MD, MBA
Department of Pathology and Department of Biomedical Informatics, University of Pittsburgh School of Medicine, University of Pittsburgh Cancer Institute, Pittsburgh, Pennsylvania

R.R. GULLAPALLI, MD, PhD
Department of Pathology, University of Pittsburgh School of Medicine, Pittsburgh, Pennsylvania

JAY L. HESS, MD, PhD, MHSA
Department of Pathology, University of Michigan Medical School, Ann Arbor, Michigan

W.A. LAFRAMBOISE, PhD
Department of Pathology and Department of Biomedical Informatics, University of Pittsburgh School of Medicine, University of Pittsburgh Cancer Institute, Pittsburgh, Pennsylvania

M. LYONS-WEILER, MS
Department of Pathology, University of Pittsburgh School of Medicine, University of Pittsburgh Cancer Institute, Pittsburgh, Pennsylvania

ZOLTÁN N. OLTVAI, MD
Associate Professor, Department of Pathology, University of Pittsburgh Medical Center, Pittsburgh, Pennsylvania

LIRON PANTANOWITZ, MD
Division of Pathology Informatics, Department of Pathology, UPMC Shadyside Hospital, University of Pittsburgh Medical Center, Pittsburgh, Pennsylvania

SEUNG PARK, MD
Division of Pathology Informatics, Department of Pathology, UPMC Shadyside Hospital, University of Pittsburgh Medical Center, Pittsburgh, Pennsylvania

ANIL VASDEV PARWANI, MD, PhD
Division of Pathology Informatics, Department of Pathology, UPMC Shadyside Hospital, University of Pittsburgh Medical Center, Pittsburgh, Pennsylvania

ROBERT J. PENNY, MD, PhD
Department of Pathology, University of Michigan Medical School, Ann Arbor, Michigan; International Genomics Consortium, Phoenix, Arizona

P. PETROSKO, MS
Department of Pathology, University of Pittsburgh School of Medicine, University of Pittsburgh Cancer Institute, Pittsburgh, Pennsylvania

DANIEL ROBINSON, PhD
Department of Pathology, Michigan Center for Translational Pathology, University of Michigan Medical School, Ann Arbor, Michigan

BRIAN R. SMITH, MD
Professor and Chair, Department of Laboratory Medicine, Yale University School of Medicine, New Haven, Connecticut

CHARLES M. STROM, MD, PhD, FAACP, FACMG, HCLD, CQ (NY), Cert Dir (CA), diplomate ABMG(CG, CBCG, CMG)
Senior Medical Director, Genetics, Quest Diagnostics Nichols Institute, San Juan Capistrano, California

SCOTT TOMLINS, MD, PhD
Department of Pathology, Michigan Center for Translational Pathology, University of Michigan Medical School, Ann Arbor, Michigan

ALAN WELLS, MD
Professor and Vice Chair, Department of Pathology, University of Pittsburgh Medical Center, Pittsburgh, Pennsylvania

JAMES M. ZIAI, MD
Departments of Pathology & Laboratory Medicine, Yale University School of Medicine, New Haven, Connecticut

Contents

Advances in computing speed and power have made a pure digital work flow for pathology. New technologies such as whole slide imaging (WSI), multispectral image analysis, and algorithmic image searching seem poised to fundamentally change the way in which pathology is practiced. This article provides the practicing pathologist with a primer on digital imaging. Building on this primer, the current state of the art concerning digital imaging in pathology is described. Emphasis is placed on WSI and its ramifications, showing how it is useful in both anatomic (histology, cytopathology) and clinical (hematopathology) pathology. Future trends are also extrapolated.

Recent advances in next-generation sequencing (NGS) methods and technology have substantially reduced costs and operational complexity leading to production of benchtop sequencers and commercial software solutions for implementation in small research and clinical laboratories. This article addresses requirements and limitations to successful implementation of these systems, including (1) calibration and validation of the instrumentation, experimental paradigm, and primary readout, (2) secure data transfer, storage, and secondary processing, (3) implementation of software tools for targeted analysis, and (4) training of research and clinical personnel to evaluate data fidelity and interpret the molecular significance of the genomic output.

New technologies, analytic techniques, and computer-assisted diagnosis algorithms will change the way pathologists and clinicians interact with and use clinical data. Simultaneously, the artisanal nature of the culture and clinical practice of medicine have made them resistant to change. An understanding of workflow science will help pathologists prepare for the changes that lie ahead in anatomic and clinical pathology, better care for patients, and make better and more respectful use of existing human and other resources. This article provides a primer on workflow science, including historical perspective, review of current literature, and extrapolation of future trends.

CLINICS IN LABORATORY MEDICINE

Preface

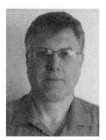

Zoltán N. Oltvai, MD
Guest Editor

There is an ongoing technological revolution marrying integrative computer technology to existing disciplines in the world that permeates all aspects of the economy, including health care. This wave of changes is now starting to affect both Anatomic and Clinical Pathology/Laboratory Medicine, developing to the point where the distinction between the two disciplines is increasingly blurred.

There are two main reasons for this technological revolution: one is due to an ongoing *hardware revolution* that entails the development of increasingly sophisticated machines that allow sample processing and analysis in previously unprecedented modes, from digital imaging pathology to nextgen sequencing and beyond.

The other reason is an ongoing *process revolution* that is deeply intertwined with contemporary advances in information technology.[1] The key change here is that processes that once took place among human beings are now being increasingly executed automatically. They are taking place in an unseen domain that is strictly digital, and that has already created a huge, and largely invisible, second economy. In health care it manifests itself today mostly in the increasingly interconnected information systems within and between medical centers and private practices, but will also increasingly affect both pathology workflow and data analysis.

Some of these changes have happened before, most evidently by the appearance of the automated clinical chemistry lab some 30 years ago. What we witness now, however, is a disruptive (re)appearance of the same trend in the whole of Anatomic Pathology and Laboratory Medicine and to a much deeper level than before. Besides the benefits of these changes, they also represent significant challenges for both the academic and the private pathologist community.

Therefore, the aim of the articles in this issue of the *Clinics in Laboratory Medicine* is to provide an overview of how the larger hardware and process revolution is impacting the whole of pathology, and how the community should prepare itself for the coming storm. In the first section (Technological and process advances), articles describe some of the new hardware platforms that will soon transform cell- and tissue-based diagnostics in anatomic and clinical pathology. They also examine how workflow

Clin Lab Med 32 (2012) ix–x
http://dx.doi.org/10.1016/j.cll.2012.07.007
labmed.theclinics.com

reorganization, modern -omic approaches, modeling, and diagnostic decision support will transform pathology. The second section (Educational, practice, and business needs) examines the required changes that will need to take place in resident and fellow training, as well as in the continuing medical education of practicing pathologists. It also envisions the future day-to-day practice of pathology. Finally, it will assess—in the context of a pathologist's career history—the changing relationships between commercial entities and academic medical centers and whether and how smaller private pathology practices can remain competitive in this unfamiliar new practice landscape.

There are a number of other topics that we could have covered in this issue, such as data storage and retrieval issues or various other emerging -omic technologies (that have been covered in part in other recent *Clinics* issues). However, in designing the content of this issue we did not seek to be comprehensive; rather we wished to provide a broader overview that vividly illustrates the coming changes while focusing on those practice aspects that have already been implemented at select institutions. We hope that such a canvas will help both our colleagues and our trainees to start to prepare for this exciting, new world of pathology in the digital age.

Alan Wells, MD
Department of Pathology
University of Pittsburgh
Pittsburgh, PA 15261, USA

Zoltán N. Oltvai, MD
Department of Pathology
University of Pittsburgh
Pittsburgh, PA 15261, USA

E-mail addresses:
wellsa@upmc.edu (A. Wells)
oltvai@pitt.edu (Z.N. Oltvai)

REFERENCE

1. Arthur WB. The second economy. McKinsey Quarterly, October 2011.

Digital Imaging in Pathology

Seung Park, MD*, Liron Pantanowitz, MD,
Anil Vasdev Parwani, MD, PhD

KEYWORDS

- Whole slide imaging • Laboratory information systems • Image analysis • Cytology
- Hematopathology • Robotic microscopy • Telepathology • Pathology 2.0

KEY POINTS

- We are about to make the leap to a pure digital work flow in pathology, so it is necessary for the practicing pathologist to understand the fundamentals of digital imaging.
- There are many exciting technologies on the market, including whole slide imaging scanners (eg, Aperio ScanScope XT [Vista, CA, USA]) and automated hematology analyzers with built-in whole slide imaging functionality (eg, CellaVision DM1200 [Palm Beach Garden, FL, USA]), but standardization and plug-and-play capability are elusive.
- Digital images have a 4-stage life cycle: acquisition, storage, manipulation, and sharing. Understanding this life cycle is key for the practicing pathologist.
- There are 3 major types of digital microscopy: static digital microscopy, robotic digital microscopy, and whole slide imaging. Each type has its pros and cons.
- Image analysis shows promise for the future, but more research is required before true frontline use is possible.

INTRODUCTION

We live in a world of infinite resolution and infinite color, limited only by the operating characteristics of our inbuilt vision-sensing system. This system is said to be unable to perceive objects less than $1/300$ in^2 in size, or resolve more than 100,000 colors in total. Although advances in technology over the past 40 years have allowed for increasingly sophisticated computer-based imaging, widespread availability of equipment with display capabilities matching or even exceeding the resolving power of the human visual processing apparatus is a recent phenomenon.[1]

This fact perhaps explains why radiologists have been quicker to adopt digital imaging–based approaches to diagnostic work flow than have pathologists. Radiologic images (even those considered high resolution) are limited by the resolving

The authors have no relationships (financial, commercial, or otherwise) to disclose.
Division of Pathology Informatics, Department of Pathology, UPMC Shadyside Hospital, University of Pittsburgh Medical Center, Suite 201, 5150 Centre Avenue, Pittsburgh, PA 15232, USA
* Corresponding author.
E-mail address: parks3@upmc.edu

Clin Lab Med 32 (2012) 557–584
http://dx.doi.org/10.1016/j.cll.2012.07.006   labmed.theclinics.com
0272-2712/12/$ – see front matter © 2012 Elsevier Inc. All rights reserved.

power of radiologic devices as opposed to the resolving power of the human eye, and are small. All radiologic images use a narrow subset of color, usually operating in 256 shades of gray; this allows them to be efficient from a computational standpoint. A fully digital work flow for radiology has been technically possible for about 30 years, and has been standard practice for at least the last decade.

Compare this situation with the practice of pathology: in our discipline, we use precision optics to magnify stained sections of tissue hundreds to thousands of times over. Because they are tissue, and not photographic representations of tissue, the resolution of our specimens is technically infinite, and limited only by the performance of our eyes. We deal with a full range of color, as opposed to the limited color palette of radiology. The process of digitally capturing and displaying even the contents of a single glass slide is more difficult than the analogous process for even the most computationally demanding radiologic study, and requires the use of exponentially greater processing power. It has therefore not been until recently that an all-digital work flow for pathology has been technically possible, and most clinical laboratories worldwide had not yet switched over to such a work flow as of the writing of this article.[2]

We therefore find ourselves at a crossroads: although current systems for digital imaging in pathology are technically complex and not easily managed by the average practicing pathologist, digital pathology will be standard practice in the future. The pathologist of tomorrow may look on our era in the same way that we look at the early 1900s and the emergence of the automobile: as a time of both great technological success and failure, with ambitious yet highly cumbersome efforts giving rise over the years to more powerful machines that are so simple that they can be easily operated by most potential users. Nevertheless, we have not yet arrived at this end point. The practicing pathologist is well served by having a general knowledge in the fundamentals of imaging technology.

IMAGING FUNDAMENTALS

Computer graphics can be broadly divided into 2 types: two-dimensional (2D) and three-dimensional (3D). 2D graphics are used in most clinical applications, although some radiologic tests (eg, positron emission tomography [PET] computed tomography [CT]) are beginning to incorporate 3D graphics for easier visualization. 2D graphics can be further subdivided into 2 models: raster and vector. The raster model is a low-level approach that approximates the way that the eye gathers image data; the fundamental graphical unit in this approach is a small square known as a picture element (pixel for short) (**Fig. 1**). Pixels are arranged in columns and rows, with the pixel resolution of any given image being expressed in 1 of 3 ways:

- Columns × rows
  - Most common and most precise way of denoting pixel resolution
  - Example: 1920 × 1080 = 1920 columns and 1080 rows of pixels
- Megapixels
  - Common in the photographic world
  - Calculated by multiplying the column and row count of the image (or screen) together and then dividing by 1,000,000
  - Example: 1920 × 1080 = 2.0736 megapixels
- Graphics array notation
  - Industry shorthand for specific columns × rows measurements
  - Commonly used to describe the pixel resolution of monitors
  - Example: 1920 × 1080 = full high definition (FHD)

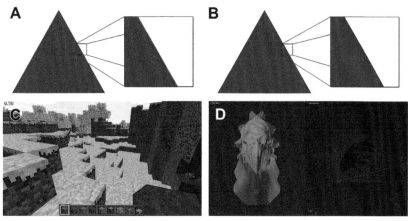

Fig. 1. Image models. (*A*) A raster image. The inset shows high magnification of one of the edges of the triangle, allowing us to visualize the individual pixels that make up this edge. (*B*) A vector image. The inset shows high magnification of one of the edges of the triangle, allowing us to see that because vector images are mathematical constructs, there is no loss of quality (and no pixels) even when highly zoomed in. (*C*) A screenshot of the video game *Minecraft*, which uses voxel-based rendering. Notice that each block is made up of smaller single-color cubes; these are the voxels. (*D*) A textured 3D model, with a view of the raw 3D mesh on the right. Notice that the mesh is made up of purely geometric shapes. (*Courtesy of* Mojang [*C*], BgDM [*D*]; with permission.)

The raw data of a pixel consist of a single binary number. The length of this number (the bit depth) is the same for all the pixels in a given image or screen (for instance, in a 24-bit image, each pixel is a 24-bit-long binary number), and the value of this number encodes for a specific color. The color that corresponds to a specific binary number can vary widely depending on the color system in use.

The raster model has 3 major advantages: (1) raster images with similar pixel resolution and bit depth have nearly identical performance characteristics, no matter how simple or complex the images are, (2) because it mimics the way the retinal pigmented epithelium processes vision, the raster model is ideally suited for extremely complex images (eg, histologic sections of tissue), and (3) most available imaging hardware uses this model. Disadvantages of this model largely relate to its fixed nature: because the bit depth and pixel resolution are defined at the time of image generation, it is impossible to later increase those parameters and expect a gain in resultant quality. On the other hand, decreasing bit depth or pixel resolution is entirely possible, but to do this is to permanently decrease the quality of the resultant image.

In comparison, the vector model is a higher-level approach, which approximates the way the brain processes raw image data, recognizing and categorizing objects in the field of view as shapes and structures (see **Fig. 1**). In this model, the fundamental graphical unit is known as a primitive, and consists of a line or a curve (from which can be derived ellipses, polygons, and mixed structures). Vector graphics are therefore completely mathematical in nature, with the raw data of vector images consisting of commands to draw certain geometric shapes of specific colors at particular positions relative to each other. The advantages of this model largely relate to its purely mathematical nature: images can be scaled up and down at will without any loss of image quality, and for simple images composed of few primitives (eg, a black triangle), file sizes and required processor power are small. The disadvantages of this model also relate to its purely mathematical nature: as an image becomes visually more complex, at some point it becomes computationally prohibitive to represent it as a set of primitives. A source raster image cannot be easily converted to a vector image, but the opposite conversion is simple. Because most monitors and printers in the world work on the raster model, a vector image must first be temporarily rasterized to be displayed on screen or printed. This situation means that for images of greater than trivial complexity, there is a performance penalty associated with the vector model.

3D imaging is split much along the same lines as 2D imaging. The volumetric model is essentially the raster model, scaled up to 3D (see **Fig. 1**). Its fundamental graphical unit is the volumetric element (voxel for short), and it shares all the advantages and disadvantages of the 2D raster model. There is 1 additional disadvantage to this model that accounts for its current rarity: the human visual system's ability to resolve volume is nearly as high as its 2D resolving power, meaning that it rapidly becomes cost-prohibitive from both a computational and a storage standpoint to use the volumetric model as the desired fidelity of the final image. In contrast, the polygonal model shares broad similarities with the 2D vector model, in that it is largely mathematical and uses the triangle as its fundamental graphical unit. In this model, one creates a 3D mesh using triangles to closely approximate (model) the 3D appearance of a real-world object. After this is created, various 2D raster images known as textures can be layered atop the triangles to lend verisimilitude to the final product, much in the way that a real-world object can be spray-painted (see **Fig. 1**). Although the polygonal model is rare in medicine, it is the dominant model used in computer-aided design (CAD) and in videogaming. The polygonal model (and not any other model) is accelerated by modern consumer graphical processing units (GPUs). This is also the reason why, despite prevailing wisdom to the contrary, powerful GPUs are of limited benefit to the practicing pathologist.

Image Size and Image Resolution

Physical image size and image resolution are completely decoupled entities. An image that is physically 2 × 2 in size, for instance, could have an image resolution of 10 × 10 pixels, 100 × 100 pixels, 600 × 600 pixels, and so on. What is changing is not how large the image is, but how closely the pixels in that image are packed (pixel density). Pixel density is measured in pixels per inch (ppi); 10 × 10 pixels, 100 × 100 pixels, and 600 × 600 pixels at 2 × 2 in are 5 ppi, 50 ppi, and 300 ppi, respectively. Complicating the issue further is the fact that the pixel density of an image file can be different from the pixel density of the monitor on which it is being viewed. As a case in point, let us consider a 1200 × 900 pixel image at 300 ppi; this translates to 4 × 3 in in physical size. This image appears as a 4 × 3 in image only on a monitor that was likewise around 300 ppi, such as the Retina Display of an iPhone 4S (a 3.5-in diagonal monitor displaying 960 × 640 pixels at 325 ppi). On the other hand, the same image viewed on a 20-in diagonal Apple Cinema Display, which displays 1680 × 1050 pixels at around 100 ppi, appears about 3 times larger in physical size than it is.

Because physical image size and image resolution are completely decoupled, it is possible to independently change one without changing the other. The same 1200 × 900 pixel image might be specified for a physical size of 4 × 3 in (in the case of 300 ppi) or 12 × 9 in (in the case of 100 ppi), and yet the image resolution does not change. Common graphics manipulation programs such as Adobe Photoshop allow the user the arbitrarily change these variables, automatically adjusting the other variables to match. When a physical image size is increased, one can either decrease the pixel density (if image resolution remains constant) or increase the image resolution (if pixel density remains constant). In contrast, when the pixel density is increased, either the physical image size is decreased (if the image resolution remains constant) or the image resolution is increased (if physical image size remains constant). The relationship between physical image size, image resolution, and pixel density is shown in **Fig. 2**.

In general, modern computer monitors tend to hover between 90 and 150 ppi, with modern smartphone displays ranging between 150 and 325 ppi. Three hundred ppi is

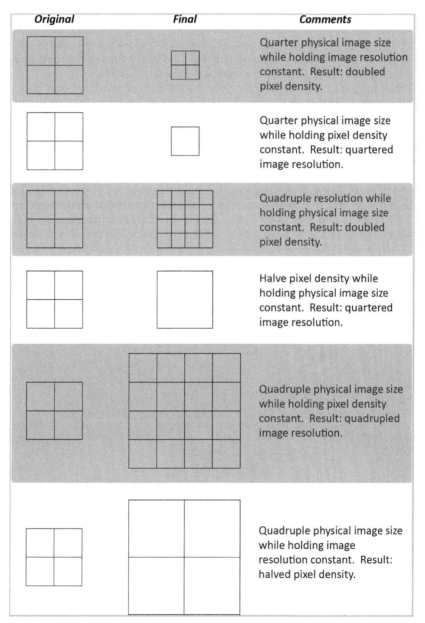

Original	Final	Comments
		Quarter physical image size while holding image resolution constant. Result: doubled pixel density.
		Quarter physical image size while holding pixel density constant. Result: quartered image resolution.
		Quadruple resolution while holding physical image size constant. Result: doubled pixel density.
		Halve pixel density while holding physical image size constant. Result: quartered image resolution.
		Quadruple physical image size while holding pixel density constant. Result: quadrupled image resolution.
		Quadruple physical image size while holding image resolution constant. Result: halved pixel density.

Fig. 2. The relationship between physical image size, image resolution, and pixel density.

said to be the limit of human detection, and is what most publishers prefer for photographs that will appear in print. Photographs less than 150 ppi are not considered fit for print, and must be reduced in physical size to compensate for lack of resolution.

Color Models

The color encoded by each individual pixel is determined by the color model of the image. Color models can be broadly subdivided into additive and subtractive flavors; additive color models begin with the absence of light and wavelengths are added until the desired color is reached, whereas subtractive color models begin with white light and wavelengths are subtracted until our desired color is reached. Although it is beyond the scope of this article to discuss every color model in depth, the practicing pathologist should be familiar with at least the 2 most common color models: red-green-blue-alpha (RGBA) and cyan-magenta-yellow-key (CMYK).

RGBA is the most common additive color model, and is the color model by which modern computer monitors operate. RGBA is simply a use of the RGB color model, but with extra (transparency/opacity) information. In RGBA (as in all additive models), 0 encodes for black and the maximum possible value encodes for white. The binary value of a pixel is subdivided into 3 or 4 channels (depending on the presence or absence of transparency data), with each channel denoting intensity of red, green, blue, or transparency (alpha). For instance, within the confines of the red channel, 0 encodes for absence of red and the maximum possible value encodes for 100% presence of pure red. All channels must be composited together to obtain a recognizable end product (**Fig. 3**). Twenty-four-bit color is interesting because 24 can be divided by both 3 and 4 (**Fig. 4**). In the case of no alpha channel, this is an 8-8-8

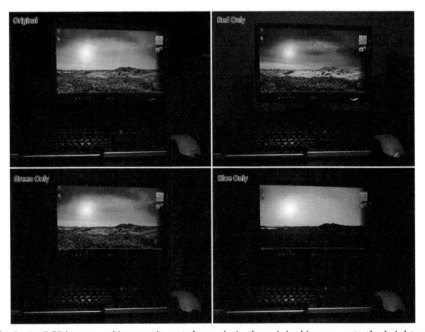

Fig. 3. An RGB image and its constituent channels. In the original image, note the bright red lights coming from the monitor power switch and the mouse, the bright green light coming from the right speaker, and the bright blue of the sky in the desktop wallpaper. Then look at the pertinent channels to see how intensity data are shown.

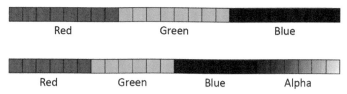

Fig. 4. 24-bit RGB versus 24-bit RGBA color.

configuration; in the case of an alpha channel, this is a 6-6-6-6 configuration. Because the bit depth is 24 in both 8-8-8 and 6-6-6-6, the total number of possible colors is the same in both cases (16.7 million). However, the 8-8-8 configuration sacrifices fine-grained variation of color for a greater coarse-grained color range, and the 6-6-6-6 configuration sacrifices coarse-grained color range for greater fine-grained variation of color.

There is a variant of RGBA that comes into play when the bit depth is 8 or less. At 8 bits and less, it is impractical to assign channels as normal, because the dynamic range of an 8-bit image is 256 colors. It becomes better to hand-pick a palette of 256 colors, explicitly assigning a color to each value. This system is known as indexed color, and it is useful in scenarios in which image clarity is paramount, but there are few colors to deal with (eg, clipart and simple Web graphics). There are several popular image file formats that use this kind of color model (see section on image compression and image files).

CMYK, on the other hand, is the most common subtractive color model. It is the color model by which modern printers operate. In CMYK, 0 encodes for white and the maximum possible value encodes for black. The binary value of a pixel is subdivided into 4 channels just as in RGBA, except in CMYK, these channels are cyan, magenta, yellow, and a fixed key color (almost always black). These channels have a 1:1 correspondence to the inks in a printer; therefore, a 0 in the cyan channel stands for "spray no cyan ink," whereas a maximum possible value in the cyan channel stands for "spray cyan ink maximally." Many publications require investigators to submit their pictures in the CMYK color model. **Fig. 5** shows the same picture as **Fig. 3**, except this time in the CMYK color model. Spend some time comparing and contrasting **Figs. 3** and **5**.

Image Compression and Image Files

The size of a digital file (image or otherwise) is expressed in bytes. One can easily calculate the size of an uncompressed digital image file using its bit depth and image resolution: file size = (pixel columns) × (pixel rows) × (bit depth)/8. Dividing by 8 is necessary because 8 bits = 1 byte. For any meaningful manipulation of an image, it must be loaded into a computer's random access memory (RAM); although at small image resolutions, this task is easily manageable, as image resolution increases, so too does the memory footprint of the image. By the time an uncompressed image file enters the gigapixel range (whole slide images commonly do this), it becomes practically unmanageable by common computer systems (**Table 1**).

Image files are commonly compressed to alleviate this problem. Compression permits image data to be stored or transmitted more efficiently. Compression refers to the act of compacting a file by removing redundant data, and comes in lossless and lossy categories. In lossless compression, no data are ever lost: when you compress then decompress a file using a lossless algorithm, the original file and the final decompressed file are identical. Compare this with lossy compression, in which

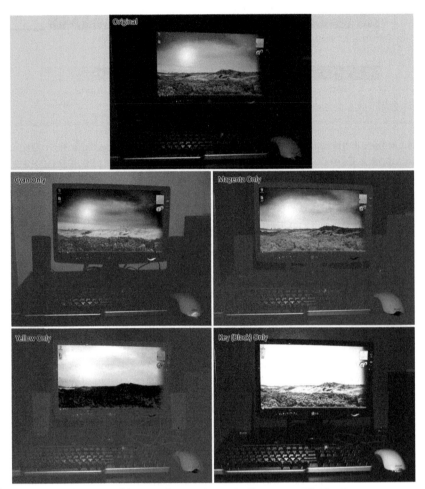

Fig. 5. A CMYK image and its constituent channels. Compare with **Fig. 6**.

Table 1
Size of uncompressed 24-bit image data

Columns × Rows	Megapixels	Size	Comments
640 × 480	0.307	0.902 MB	Common Microsoft PowerPoint slide size
800 × 600	0.480	1.373 MB	Common Microsoft PowerPoint slide size
1024 × 768	0.786	2.25 MB	Common Microsoft PowerPoint slide size
1280 × 720	0.921	2.63 MB	720 p HDTV size
1920 × 1080	2.073	5.932 MB	1080 p HDTV size
2592 × 1944	5.038	14.416 MB	Common size for smartphone cameras
2848 × 2136	6.083	17.404 MB	Common size for point-and-shoot cameras
4592 × 3056	14.033	40.149 MB	Common size for digital SLR cameras
40,000 × 40,000	1600	4.577 GB	Approximate size of a whole slide image

Abbreviations: GB, gigabytes; HDTV, high-definition television; MB, megabytes; SLR, single-lens reflex.

information is irrevocably lost during the compression phase. In general, lossless compression does not result in files as small as can be achieved by lossy compression. Because no data are ever lost, lossless compression is used in situations in which 100% fidelity of data is critical. Lossless compression is therefore found in the following applications:

- Compression of large software packages for delivery to the consumer
  - Examples: Microsoft Windows 7 and Apple Mac OS × are both compressed using lossless compression to fit into a single installation DVD
- Compression of text files and office documents
  - Example: Microsoft Word 2007 and onward use a new file format called DOCX, which at its heart is a set of eXtensible Markup Language (XML) files compressed together using a common lossless compression algorithm. The zip file format is also used for data compression and archiving.

Lossy compression, on the other hand, throws away data permanently. The smaller the desired final file, the more data are thrown away (**Fig. 6**). This characteristic usually strikes most people as a terrible idea at first glance. As noted earlier, there are many purposes for which lossy compression is entirely inappropriate. However, there is 1 domain in which the use of lossy compression has become overwhelmingly standard: audiovisual data. These kinds of data (images, sounds, music, video) are notoriously nonrepeating in nature, and cannot be losslessly compressed by more than a factor of 2 (in practice, a factor of 1.5 is common). However, audiovisual data have 1 characteristic

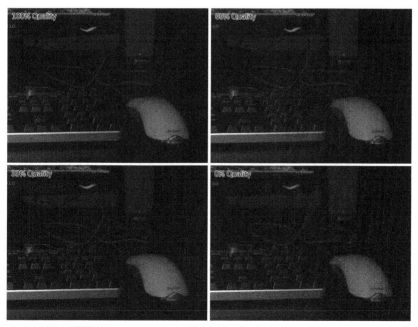

Fig. 6. An 800 × 600 image compressed with JPEG, a common lossy image compression algorithm, at 100%, 66%, 33%, and 0% quality. Uncompressed = 1393 KB; 100% quality = 291 KB; 66% quality = 84.1 KB; 33% quality = 51.7 KB; 0% quality = 33 KB. Note that there is little perceptual difference between 100% and 66% quality, even although the file size has been decreased by two-thirds. The difference between 100% and 0% quality, on the other hand, is stark.

that makes them well suited to lossy compression: the fact that human sensory systems not only have limitations, they also have compensatory mechanisms that are easily exploited.

There are several commonly used file formats (**Table 2**). Some of these (such as Bitmap [BMP]) are uncompressed. Others (such as Photoshop Document [PSD]) use lossless compression. However, the most popular formats use lossy compression. Of these formats, 6 in particular deserve deeper analysis:

- JPEG
  - Stands for Joint Picture Experts Group
  - File extension: .JPG or .JPEG
  - Color model: RGBA
  - A 24-bit lossy compression algorithm specifically designed for use with photographs
  - Ubiquitous and universally supported
  - All cameras have the ability to take photographs in JPEG

Table 2 Common image file formats		
Name	**Extension**	**Comments**
Bitmap	.BMP	An uncompressed file format with universal support, but no longer heavily used
Graphics Interchange Format	.GIF	Was once the de facto standard for small graphics on the Web
Portable Network Graphic	.PNG	A highly versatile file format that incorporates the strengths of both GIFs and BMPs
Joint Photographic Experts Group	.JPG, .JPEG	A lossy compression algorithm that is the de facto standard for photographic image files
Joint Photographic Experts Group 2000	.JP2	An advanced version of JPEG; currently not in widespread use
Tagged Image File Format	.TIF, .TIFF	A container file format that can use any color model, any compression, and can contain more than 1 image at a time
Photoshop Document	.PSD	A proprietary file format that shows the highest versatility of any existing image file format, but can be opened only in Adobe Photoshop
Camera Raw	.RAW	Raw data from the sensor of a digital camera, which must be further processed before being rendered
Postscript	.PS, .EPS	A standard file format used to send commands to printers; currently not in widespread use
Portable Document Format	.PDF	A proprietary successor to Postscript; currently the de facto standard for formatted document access on the Web
Scalable Vector Graphic	.SVG	An open standard for vector graphics (all other formats listed in this table, with the exception of PSD, are raster only) that is gaining popularity on the Web
Digital Imaging and Communication in Medicine	.DICOM	An image messaging file format that is standard in medicine; most highly used in radiology

- JPEG 2000
  - An advanced version of JPEG (likewise lossy)
  - File extension: .JP2
  - Color model: RGBA
  - More flexible than JPEG, at the cost of greater software complexity
  - Not in widespread use, except in the arena of whole slide imaging (WSI)
- PSD
  - Stands for Photoshop Document
  - File extension: .PSD
  - Color model: any
  - A proprietary, losslessly compressed file format for use with the popular graphics editing software Adobe Photoshop
  - Seamlessly combines raster and vector graphics
  - Enables nondestructive editing of graphics by usage of a layer metaphor
- TIFF
  - Stands for Tagged Image File Format
  - File extension: .TIF or .TIFF
  - Color model: any
  - A container file format that does not specify a compression algorithm at all
    - As a result, TIFFs can be completely uncompressed, be losslessly compressed, or even use lossy compression algorithms like JPEG
  - Can contain multiple images at the same time
    - WSI scanner vendors exploit this fact to package multiple magnification levels (usually compressed with JPEG 2000) in a single file
- GIF
  - Stands for Graphical Interchange Format
  - File extension: .GIF
  - Color model: indexed
  - Losslessly compresses pixel size and location, but lossily compresses (dithers) color into a 256-color palette
  - Inherently supports animation
  - Was the de facto standard on the Web for small graphics, but has now been supplanted by PNG
  - Was patent-encumbered until recently
- PNG
  - Stands for Portable Network Graphic
  - File extension: .PNG
  - Color model: RGBA or indexed
  - Similar to GIF in most respects
    - Except PNG can losslessly compress color up to 32 bits in PNG32 mode
  - Has recently become a de facto standard on the Web for small graphics, supplanting GIF

IMAGING DEVICES IN PATHOLOGY

Digital imaging has made significant inroads in our specialty, especially in anatomic pathology. Digital images can be introduced at just about any point in the laboratory work flow:

- Digital imaging is generally not used in the preanalytical phase of the laboratory test process, although it is plausible (especially in cases in which establishing

a chain of custody for the specimen is critical) that pictures could be taken during this phase for documentation purposes.
- Gross photography has long been a feature of the analytical phase, as has taking photomicrographs during sign-out. Because of increased ease of use and decreased logistical roadblocks (eg, the need to buy film is eliminated in digital imaging), digital imaging has made these activities more popular than ever.
  - With the advent of WSI technology, we are coming tantalizingly close to enabling an all-digital work flow for pathologists, much in the same way that radiologists converted to an all-digital work flow in the late 1990s.
- The postanalytical phase has traditionally been the time for activities (eg, quality assurance, teaching, and scholarly research) that are greatly enhanced by the addition of digital imaging.

Digital Cameras

Digital cameras are ubiquitous in daily life, being available in a wide variety of sizes with widely varying performance characteristics. Cameras are found either (1) as stand-alone units (compact point-and-shoot cameras; digital single-lens reflex [DSLR] cameras) or (2) integrated into other devices (mobile phones, laptops, and whole slide scanners). Cameras that are integrated into other devices tend to have fixed specifications, with optical elements that cannot be swapped at will. This characteristic leads, as a general rule, to lower performance and poorer-quality photographs. Stand-alone cameras, on the other hand, tend to be more flexible in this regard. Although point-and-shoot cameras are as monolithic as their device-integrated counterparts, they use larger, higher-quality components throughout. DSLR cameras take this feature 1 step further, offering even higher-quality components and allowing the user to swap between lenses at will. Cameras specifically designed to interface with microscopes are conceptually akin to DSLRs, in that the major optical component (the lens unit in a DSLR; the microscope in a microscope camera) can be swapped out at will. However, unlike DSLRs, these cameras generally require a dedicated connection to a host computer (with specialized control software installed) at all times. There are highly specialized digital cameras that are designed for advanced imaging purposes, such as the electron-multiplying charged couple devices (CCDs) found in electron microscopes.

At its simplest, a digital camera is made up of an optical focusing pathway (usually a lens), which directs light at a silicon chip known as a sensor. Unlike most silicon chips (which are entirely digital in nature), sensors are hybrid analog/digital designs that first gather photons, then convert them into electrical signals to later be processed into image files. Sensors are of either CCD or complementary metal oxide semiconductor (CMOS) design; CMOS designs are relatively easier to manufacture and use less power, but until recently have delivered lesser image quality compared with contemporary CCD designs. The larger the sensor, the more light it can capture and consequently the better the quality of the resultant image. Whereas in the purely digital realm, a higher pixel density is almost always a good thing, in the realm of sensors, this is not the case: given 2 sensors of the same physical size, built using the same technology but with differing pixel densities (usually expressed in megapixels), the sensor with the lower megapixel count is more sensitive to light, and capable of taking better pictures. This situation is because the more pixels you try to extract from a sensor, the smaller the individual photon-sensing sites of the sensor must be, causing a decrease in light sensitivity.

Point-and-shoot and DSLR cameras have been widely used in the clinical laboratory for the purposes of gross photography. Before the advent of dedicated gross pathology workstations with integrated cameras, these cameras were the only option to take gross photographs. Point-and-shoot cameras (eg, Casio Exilim EX-Z550) have a retractable lens and built-in flash, and are popular for their ease of use. However, their sensors are small, usually leading to less than satisfactory image quality. DSLRs (eg, Canon EOS 7D), on the other hand, offer larger sensors and interchangeable lens systems, offering professional-grade image quality at the cost of increased operating complexity and usually increased equipment delicacy. There also exist prosumer (between professional and consumer) cameras that straddle the line between point-and-shoot cameras and DSLRs. Some of them have sensors that rival DSLRs but have fixed lenses (eg, Fujifilm FinePix X100); others have smaller sensors, but feature interchangeable lens systems (eg, Panasonic Lumix GF-1). Cameras integrated on mobile phones have recently been improving in quality (eg, Nokia PureView 808). As a result, they have come into more widespread use in the clinical laboratory, primarily because of their expediency. All of these handheld cameras have also been used with a microscope for micrography, either by capturing a digital image through the eyepiece or using a microscope adaptor, with surprisingly good results (**Fig. 7**).[3,4]

Digital gross photography units can be found as stand-alone solutions or integrated into the design of grossing stations. The interesting thing about these units is not so much the camera part of the equation (usually, these are off-the-shelf DSLRs with off-the-shelf lenses) but the demanding environmental conditions under which they must work. Purpose-built shells are used to house the camera, isolating it from the operating environment. The controls (including camera movement, camera zoom, and shutter release) are made as hands-free as possible, both for easier integration into work flow and to avoid contamination with blood and other body fluids. Digital gross photography units almost always come with a host computer and an image management solution; ideally, they allow for upload of taken images directly into the laboratory information system (LIS). For more details on this issue, see the section on the digital imaging life cycle.

Dedicated microscope cameras, although not as versatile as handheld cameras, are purpose-built for photomicroscopy and as a result deliver better image quality in that application. These cameras are attached to a microscope via a C-mount adaptor and usually require a dedicated connection (USB [Universal Serial Bus] or FireWire) to a host computer with specialized control software installed. Different cameras are suitable for varying contrast methods, including light microscopy and fluorescent work. Because these units are by-and-large permanently placed, it is technically possible

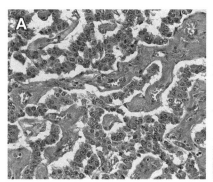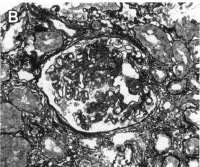

Fig. 7. Example photomicrographs taken with the camera of an Apple iPhone 4S. (*A*) Pancreatic neuroendocrine tumor (hematoxylin-eosin); (*B*) normal glomerulus (Jones Silver). (*Courtesy of* Dr Milon Amin, University of Pittsburgh Medical Center.)

to interface them via software directly to the LIS, allowing for smoother integration of photomicroscopy into the daily work flow (see the section on the digital imaging life cycle for additional details).

WSI Scanners

In the last decade, digital imaging in pathology has been completely changed by the development of WSI technology. Conventional (static) photomicrography has limitations, largely because it is possible to select only limited fields of interest and photograph them, as opposed to being able to present the entire slide with full visual fidelity. WSI solves this problem by scanning entire glass slides, outputting an image file that is a faithful digitized reproduction of the glass slide, (complete with full objective lens zooming functionality) rather than of 1 small microscopic field.

WSI scanners are best thought of as microscopes under full robotic control, attached to highly specialized cameras containing high-performance photosensors. A WSI scanner methodically captures the entire slide, field by field, and merges all the fields together into a single file often known as a virtual slide or a whole slide image (also abbreviated WSI). This situation leads to an interesting problem: individual photosensors and microscopic fields of view are not large enough to be able to take a single shot of a fully magnified slide. Many solutions to this problem have been attempted, but the 2 predominant approaches are tile-based imaging, in which a square photosensor is used to capture multiple tiles adjacent to each other, and line scan-based imaging (otherwise known as time-domain integration), in which an oblong photosensor is used to continually capture strips of image data as it sweeps through the slide (**Fig. 8**). Tile-based WSI scanners are more common than progressive scan-based WSI scanners, but both can offer excellent (and equivalent) results.

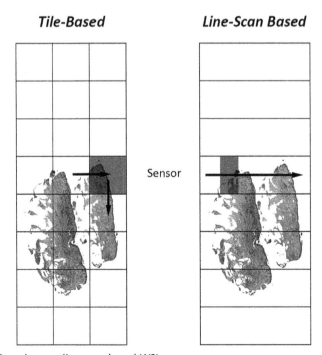

Fig. 8. Tile-based versus line scan-based WSI.

Most current scanners with slide feeders offer scan times of around 1 to 2 minutes (at 20 times).[5] The quality of focusing is limited by multiple optical and mechanical parameters, notably numerical aperture (NA) of the objective and movement resolution on the vertical (z-) axis. Higher NA causes the distance that can be resolved to become smaller, effectively increasing resolution (**Fig. 9**). All scanners come with automatic algorithms to determine the optimal focus (focal planes) throughout the slide, but most scanners have the capacity to image only 1 level of the z-axis at a time. Although this is not a problem for most general surgical pathology cases that routinely deal with 3-μm to 5-μm tissue sections, it becomes more of a critical issue in the subdiscipline of cytopathology, in which glass slides may contain thick smears or 3D cell groups, in which access to all levels of the z-axis is a must. Newer WSI scanners often integrate the capability to take multiple levels of the z-axis at once, but human intervention for optimal z-axis scanning is still the exception rather than the rule. The adoption of WSI in areas like cytopathology and hematopathology has been slower than its use in general surgical pathology.[6]

WSI file formats

WSI files have the capacity to be exponentially larger than other digital images used in health care. Also, unlike conventional digital image files (which typically contain a single image view at a single resolution), WSI files are usually formatted as multiresolution

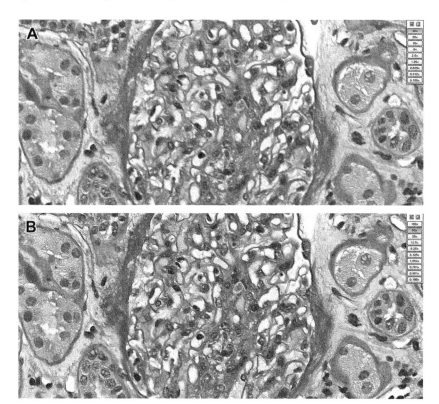

Fig. 9. How NA affects resolution. (*A*) Scan at .75 NA; (*B*) scan at .95 NA. Note that the scan at .95 NA is sharper than the scan at .75 NA. This difference is because the scan at .95 NA has greater resolution than the scan at .75 NA. (*Courtesy of* Andrew Lesniak, University of Pittsburgh Medical Center.)

pyramids that contain multiple images comprising multiple magnifications (**Fig. 10**). The base TIFF file format is often used by vendors because multiple images must fit into 1 image file, usually using high JPEG2000-based lossy compression. Every vendor has its own proprietary file format, and although there has been work in DICOM (digital imaging and communication in medicine) supplements 122 and 124 toward a universal

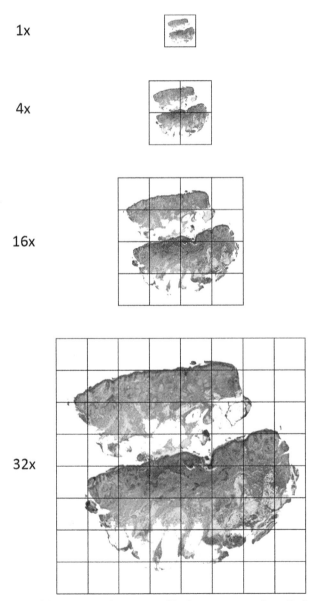

Fig. 10. The pyramidal structure of most WSI file formats. Note that all tiles (denoted as squares in this diagram) are usually stored in the same file as separate images, meaning that a file format such as TIFF becomes necessary to hold the (usually) thousands of images that comprise a single WSI.

interchange standard, it has been left to the vendors to implement true interoperability. As a result, it is currently impossible to read 1 vendor's WSI files using another vendor's viewer. Open-source efforts (such as OpenSlide [http://www.opendp.org/]) exist to attempt to bridge this compatibility gap, but so far a truly universal WSI file format standard has not yet been developed.[7]

GPUs

GPUs are found in all modern computers, and are used for displaying images. At one point, GPUs displayed only characters and a limited number of colors on a computer screen. Subsequently, 3D modeling became increasingly important, and the video-game industry became the major driver of progress in computer graphics. GPUs have now become specialized units that can run demanding calculations at speeds 1000 times faster than general-purpose computer processors.

Despite the popular notion that you need a powerful graphics card to perform demanding image analysis, in pathology informatics, this is not yet the case. Routine image processing using current computer systems tends to use only the central processing unit and uses the GPU only to draw what appears on the screen. However, this situation is changing; interest has been growing in the use of the increasingly sophisticated GPUs as fast general-purpose processors for certain classes of calculations. It is perhaps only a matter of time until GPU-accelerated image analysis becomes the rule rather than the exception in pathology, and when that time comes the pathologist will require a GPU that is powerful enough to easily run programs with image-processing algorithms written in GPU-accelerated programming languages such as OpenCL.[8]

Monitors

GPUs require computer monitors (or electronic visual display units) for output visualization. These monitors come in all shapes and sizes, with a wide array of parameters (**Table 3**). In the past, cathode ray tube (CRT)-based displays, which use technologies similar to those found in old televisions, were dominant. By 2004 (when CRTs became largely obsolete), they were known to have excellent color reproduction and viewing angles, but accepted only analog input and were large and heavy. Liquid crystal display (LCD) technology (with thin, light, digital displays), has replaced CRT technology, except in highly specialized environments. LCDs are more compact (thin), light, have lower power consumption, and are available in more varied sizes or shapes. However, LCDs have some limitations related to viewing angles and brightness distortion. Several kinds of LCD monitors are available, each with advantages and disadvantages. Early laptops used monochrome passive-matrix LCDs. High-resolution LCD computer monitors and televisions use an active matrix structure. Four common LCD types are listed as follows:

- Twisted nematic (TN): the most common LCD type. These LCDs are fast and cheap, but suffer from poor color reproduction and limited viewing angles (**Fig. 11**).
- In-plane switching (IPS): has good color reproduction and the best viewing angles of any current LCD technology, but their response times are not as fast as TN panels. They are also more expensive than TN technology, being widely used in high-end professional monitors (see **Fig. 11**).
- Patterned vertical alignment (PVA): this has good color reproduction and good viewing angles. It has faster response times than IPS monitors, but is rare compared with IPS technology, and usually found in high-end professional monitors.

Table 3
Monitor performance parameters

Parameter	Measurement
Monitor size	Measured diagonally in inches
Display resolution	Number of distinct pixels in each dimension that can be displayed
Aspect ratio	Ratio of horizontal to vertical length (4:3, 16:10, and 16:9 are all standard)
Luminance	Measured in candelas per square meter (cd/m^2; also referred to as a nit)
Dot pitch	Distance between subpixels of the same color in millimeters
Refresh rate	Number of times in a second that the display is illuminated (measured in Hz)
Response time	Time that a pixel takes to go from active to inactive and back to active again, measured in milliseconds
Contrast ratio	Ratio of the luminosity of the brightest color to that of the darkest color
Power consumption	Measured in watts
Viewing angle	Maximum angle at which images on the monitor can be viewed, without excessive degradation to the image, measured in degrees horizontally and vertically
LCD technology	The way the liquid crystals are laid out and function (twisted nematic, in-plane switching, vertical alignment, active matrix organic light-emitting diode); highly influences all of the above parameters

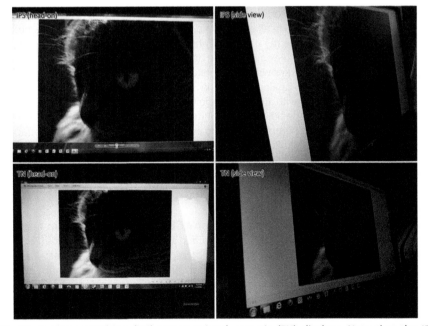

Fig. 11. In-plane switching (IPS) versus twisted nematic (TN) displays. Note that the IPS display faithfully renders color no matter what the viewing angle, as opposed to the TN display, which displays color inversion at angles that are not orthogonal to the monitor.

- Active matrix organic light-emitting diode (AMOLED): these LCDs offer good color reproduction and good viewing angles. They have the potential to use less power than any other LCD monitor type, and are thus often used in mobile devices. However, the organic elements in this technology degrade over time, giving AMOLEDs a finite life span.

Although it is probably best that pathologists should work with good high-resolution IPS or PVA monitors and avoid TN monitors, best-case parameters for work with WSI have yet to be completely established. The topic of optimal display characteristics has been well studied, but almost all of these studies were in radiology, which has different demands in terms of imaging devices from those of digital pathology. Several studies are under way to gauge the most important monitor parameters for use by pathologists.

THE DIGITAL IMAGING LIFE CYCLE

Traditionally, nondigital photography (Polaroids, Kodachromes) has been used in both gross and microscopic pathology for diagnostic and teaching purposes. This kind of usage has extended itself naturally into the digital realm, with many practices exclusively using digital cameras to take pictures of gross and microscopic specimens. However, as digital photography has become more prevalent, it is becoming necessary for there to be some way to manage the growing repository of digital imaging data. In order to understand how digital images can be managed and used within the pathology work flow, it is necessary to understand the digital imaging life cycle: image acquisition, storage, manipulation, and sharing.

Acquisition

Acquisition refers to the process of creating the digital image, with a digital camera or WSI scanner. Although some interchange standards (eg, TWAIN) exist that can facilitate this process, it is by no means plug-and-play. Not many pieces of imaging hardware and software (and almost no WSI scanners) are integrated with LIS software; this is problematic because an end user is more likely to take (and integrate into reporting) photographs if the functionality to quickly take a snapshot of the relevant case is available within the work flow of the LIS itself, rather than the alternative (in which the end user has to go to a separate application to take the image, save it, and then import it into the LIS).

Storage

Storage refers to the specific manner in which the digital image is stored, both on physical media and in the database of the LIS or a separate repository. Hence, there are 2 approaches to consider: an image management module as an integral part of the LIS, or a separate image management system that manually or ideally automatically feeds images into the LIS (**Fig. 12**). Both approaches have their advantages and disadvantages.

Integral image management within the LIS means that the user never has to leave the LIS and (perhaps more importantly) that the image can be more easily manipulated in the setting of the LIS. Images can be kept in a gallery for internal use (eg, documentation purposes), or embedded into final reports. At the time of acquisition, the LIS can also record image metadata into its database, including but not limited to the date the picture was taken, the location where the picture was taken, and the user who took the picture. Disadvantages of this approach include: (1) the user requires access to the LIS; (2) image editing and sharing tools are restricted to what the LIS explicitly supports (either as native tools or through a TWAIN interface); (3) it is more difficult for the end user to directly access the raw image data; (4) if the LIS goes down, so

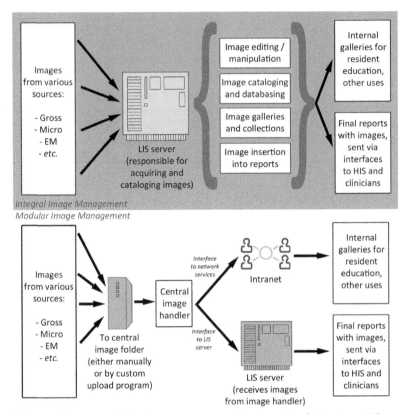

Fig. 12. Integral versus modular image management systems in relation to an LIS.

too do all digital images in the system; and (5) the file format in which the images are stored may be proprietary, hindering interoperability.

Modular image management can accomplish everything that integral image management can, but through different means. In this system, images are conglomerated (either explicitly by individual end users or through a customized image upload program) into a single central image repository, from where they can be manually imported into the LIS or use an automated image-processing program to send the images to various end points (eg, into the LIS, into internal image galleries for teaching purposes). The main advantages of this approach have to do with flexibility; the user does not need to first get into the LIS and they can use any image-editing or image-sharing software desired. Image acquisition capabilities need not be integrated into the LIS, removing the problem that "We don't support this hardware/software yet." The file formats used in this schema are generally universally readable, reducing vendor lock-in. Modular image management introduces the additional overhead of having to administer an entirely different system, and the fact that certain kinds of data about the image may not be readily available to the LIS.[9]

Manipulation

Manipulation refers to how an image might be annotated or further transformed by image-editing software. Some LISs provide basic image-editing modules, with support for frequently used functions like inserting measurements or captions. The modular image management model has a wider choice of image editors (eg, Adobe Photoshop) to accomplish the same thing. When such changes are made, there are 2 ways to store them: (1) as annotation layers/separate files that do not alter the underlying image data but that cannot be read except by the image management system, or (2) as universally readable flat images that have the annotation elements burned onto them (thus destroying the underlying image data).

Sharing

The main form of sharing in LIS image management is the integration of images into the final report. Other forms of sharing include the use of images in consultation, education, or as adjuncts to tumor board presentations. This sharing is more easily accomplished through a modular image management system, but all existing integral image management systems have import/export capabilities. Embedding images in pathology reports is a growing trend among pathology practices, with obvious benefits: (1) added documentation to reports, (2) value-added reports for marketing, and (3) facilitation of teaching and communication to patients and clinicians. However, critics of this practice point out that work flow interruption caused by taking and inserting images is not reimbursed, and that the legal liability for embedding images in pathology reports is not well understood.[10]

The Digital Cockpit for Pathology Sign-Out

As WSI (and with it, a pure digital work flow for pathologists) becomes more prevalent, it is likely that we will see the LIS integrating additional image management features, especially with relation to the rich metadata that can be embedded in these large image sets. However, in order for a pure digital work flow to become a reality in pathology, there is an important user interface problem that LISs have to surmount first: the concept of the digital cockpit.

As any pathologist knows, it is impossible to truly sign out a glass slide in isolation. Relevant case data (including clinical data, the gross report and its associated images, and older pathology reports from the same patient) are often crucial in the delivery of the correct diagnosis. Traditionally, this diagnosis has involved multiple sets of glass slides and multiple pieces of paper for the pathologist to keep track of. The need to manage and keep track of this information is not lessened by the addition of an all-digital work flow: such a work flow only emphasizes that the image data by itself is not enough.

There is growing interest in the specific way that an LIS might present the available data on a case to the pathologist. This is a difficult problem with user interfaces, and most current solutions rely on at least 2 monitors (one to display the WSI, the other to display case and clinical data) for information display purposes. It is not known what form the optimal digital cockpit for pathology will take, but given the history of the LIS, imaging systems, and adoption of mobile computing in medicine, we are confident that it will likely only happen with full participation from practicing pathologists in collaboration with user interface researchers and vendors.

DIGITAL MICROSCOPY

There are 3 kinds of digital microscopy in widespread use; each one has its advantages and disadvantages. Static digital microscopy is the oldest, the simplest, and still the most dominant form of digital microscopy. Robotic digital microscopy requires the most complexity in mechanical design and is best suited to rapid telepathology applications, such as frozen sections. The technical aspects of WSI were briefly discussed in the section on whole slide imaging scanners; this section focuses on the application of WSI. There is significant overlap between these kinds of digital microscopy: for instance, a whole slide image can be used to create static digital micrographs, and some devices have both robotic digital microscopy and WSI capabilities.

Static Digital Microscopy

Static digital microscopy refers to the act of taking still digital photomicrographs (snapshots). With the exception that the equipment being used is digital in nature, this is no different from the traditional approach of taking photographs and Kodachromes of interesting fields of view. This is the form of microscopy that is currently used for paper publications, and its integration is becoming increasingly common in surgical pathology reports. The need for long-distance hematopathologic consultation in low-resource areas (combined with the increased ubiquity of smartphones with powerful telecommunication hardware and relatively high-quality built-in cameras) has resulted in the development of smartphone telehematopathology. This application has been shown to be effective in at least limited case reports, and is an ingenious way of using low-cost technology to positively affect clinical care of patients.[3,4]

Advantages of static digital microscopy include:

- Simplicity
- Intuitive to most pathologists
- Lowest start-up and maintenance costs for equipment
- Highly amenable to paper publication
- Small file sizes that are easy to store and transmit forward

Disadvantages of static digital microscopy include:

- The ability to only select 1 field of view and plane of focus at a time
- Digital photomicrographs may not be representative of the true disease process
- Wide variability in photographic quality depending on the skill of the user
- Telepathology is dependent on the person taking the photograph

Although static digital microscopy is appropriate for simple uses, it is generally not a good modality for primary diagnosis, consultation, image analysis, or any other use case in which access to the full slide is critical. Because of its advantages and its current ubiquity, it is not likely that this form of digital microscopy will ever become fully obsolete.

Robotic Digital Microscopy

Robotic digital microscopy entails a robotic microscope attached to a microscope camera that can be viewed live from other computers. Originally developed to allow telepathology for time-critical applications such as frozen sections, robotic digital microscopes almost always integrate a WSI scanner, making them hybrid devices capable of operating in both live and WSI modes. There are many network considerations related to the usage of these devices, because a high-quality live video stream from a robotic digital microscope can be resource-intensive to encode and bandwidth-intensive to broadcast on a real-time basis. Moreover, firewalls are notorious for blocking certain remote signals intended to control microscope robotics. Many of these devices enable telepathology by the use of third-party screen-sharing software, which can add even further to latency as perceived by the end user and raise security concerns. Most vendors of these telepathology solutions are moving toward using Web 2.0 technologies to allow direct access to and control of the live photomicrographic feed on a real-time basis, but this has not yet become widespread.[11]

Advantages of robotic digital microscopy include:

- Access to the entire slide
- User controls the microscope and the image
- Good image quality
- Fast (but not immediate) driving speed
- Viewed areas can be tracked (audit trail)

Disadvantages of robotic digital microscopy include:

- Need for a highly experienced host (assistant)
- Expensive
- Slow (approximately 10 minutes/slide)
- Both host and recipient require integrated software
- Static image capture may not be included with software
- Lack of interoperability between different manufacturers
- High bandwidth requirements
- Need to support and maintain older technology

WSI

The development of automated, high-speed, high-resolution WSI has had a significant effect on education, quality assurance, research, image analysis, second-opinion consultations, and primary clinical diagnosis. Education is a clear-cut use case for WSI, because a single representative slide set can be digitized for use by all students, as opposed to having to cut separate slide sets for each individual. Lost and damaged slides become a thing of the past, and the ability to annotate slides on a real-time basis has led to innovative and interactive uses of WSI in medical education. For instance, one institution has used Web 2.0 technologies to enable collaborative virtual microscopy for all medical students taking its M2-year pathology course; this technology has been embraced by the students, and is now a standard part of the curriculum at that institution.[12]

Quality assurance is also greatly facilitated by use of WSI. Digitized slides made readily available to pathologists in the LIS or on a network can be used for several quality assurance tasks, including teleconsultation, gauging both interobserver and intraobserver variance, proficiency testing, and archiving of slides. For example, the College of American Pathologists now optionally sends WSIs in addition to glass slides of certain proficiency testing cases.[13]

WSI has seen widespread use in research, especially in the arena of experimental image analysis. Because advanced WSI scanners are able to work in both transmitted light and fluorescent modes, it is possible to use WSI for experiments involving immunohistochemistry, immunofluorescence, and fluorescence in-situ hybridization. WSI has also found a home in tissue microarrays (TMAs), a high-throughput technology for rapid analysis of protein expression across hundreds of patient samples. Many databases storing experimental TMA data have begun to integrate TMA WSIs directly into their data sets, unlocking techniques for rapid visualization and algorithmic image analysis.[14]

Advantages of WSI include:

- Access to the entire slide
- Automated scanning is possible
- High resolution of images
- Ability for simultaneous viewing of images
- Effective for education

- Audit trail is possible
- Added software available (eg, teleconferencing, image management, and analysis)

Disadvantages of WSI include:

- High start-up and maintenance costs
- Not all slides are amenable to automatic scanning
- High bandwidth requirements
- Large (multiple gigabyte) file sizes
- Better at present for histology than cytology or hematopathology
- Poor vendor interoperability

WSI, primary diagnosis, regulatory issues, and validation

The tale of WSI in primary diagnosis has been a tale of hope, frustration, and regulatory woe (perhaps in that order). It is technically feasible to use WSI for routine pathologic diagnosis if the images are at all times an accurate representation of the scanned glass slide. Several studies have shown that when those conditions are met, there is little to no difference between a diagnosis rendered via WSI as opposed to one rendered via conventional microscopy with a glass slide.[15–17] Some investigators note that a review of a WSI took participants longer than a review of a glass slide, whereas others note that WSI without z-stacking is not appropriate for cytopathology and hematopathology.[16] Nevertheless, some pathology laboratories (eg, notably the general pathology laboratory at Kalmar County Hospital in Kalmar, Sweden) have gone fully digital, rendering routine pathologic diagnosis using WSI only.

The advantages of using WSI in this way are immediately apparent: portability, ease of sharing, and retrieval of archival images, and the ability to make use of computer-aided image analysis tools. WSI has benefits for remote consultation, eliminating the need for glass slides to be physically mailed from one location to another. Consultation can instead occur in real time across the Internet, with both the primary and consulting pathologist benefiting from this increased communication. However, formidable barriers (such as technical difficulty, lack of a true digital cockpit for sign-out, lack of truly standardized WSI file formats, justification of the added costs, and the need to train practicing pathologists in optimal use of new technology) also exist.

The US Food and Drug Administration (FDA) has recently declared WSI systems as class III medical devices. Before this announcement, many companies that market a WSI system had hoped that the FDA would declare WSI systems as class II (moderate risk devices that already have a predicate device on the market) or as class I (no premarket notification required). The FDA uses the class III categorization to label devices as highest risk. Class III devices are therefore the most highly regulated of all medical devices, requiring not only general controls (eg, quality system regulation and good manufacturing procedures) but also premarket approval. In light of this situation, individual WSI systems now have to be rigorously validated for every intended use, and it is not yet known how narrow or broad an intended use can be. These validation studies may be too expensive and too difficult for smaller companies to perform, and even for companies that have the resources to perform these studies, a large amount of time will be necessary. It is estimated, therefore, that we are at least 5 years away from the inception of the first FDA-approved WSI systems for primary diagnosis.

In the meantime, efforts by both industry and academia to deal with the issue of WSI validation are ongoing. On the industry side, corporations like Aperio and Omnyx lead the charge in device validation. On the side of academia, the College of American Pathologists (CAP) has created a work group on WSI validation, which has recently drafted 13 recommendations for laboratories to follow if they want to validate WSI systems. Although the CAP has no accreditation program checklists for WSI validation, these draft statements are a move in that direction.[18,19]

WSI in hematopathology

Although most uses of WSI are found in anatomic pathology, there are several devices that use WSI technology in hematopathology. These devices (eg, the CellaVision DM1200 [**Fig. 13**] and Bloodhound Integrated Hematology System) combine automated smear preparation, cell counting, and cell sorting with full-fledged use of WSI to deliver intriguing integrated solutions that allow for rapid visualization and verification of tests like blood differential counts. Because a WSI is created for every smear, the full benefit of WSI technology in applications such as telehematopathology, consultation, education, quality assurance, and research can be unlocked. The Cella-Vision DM1200 was FDA approved in 2009, whereas the Bloodhound has not yet been FDA approved. It seems likely that more devices of this type will be developed and brought to market in the future.[20]

IMAGE ANALYSIS

Although we have used combinations of immunohistochemical stains to assist in diagnostic purposes for decades, it has not been until recently that we have been able to use computer algorithms to automatically score immunohistochemical studies. Historically, important analytical measurements such as cell counting and staining intensity quantification have been impossible to perform reliably with traditional approaches; however, automated computer-based techniques can render these measurements trivial to perform and with greater accuracy and reproducibility.

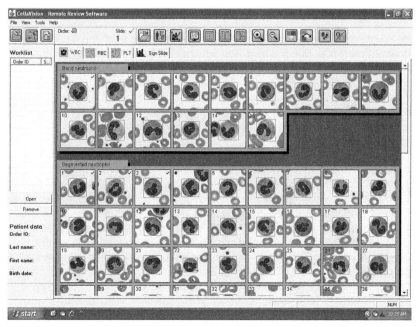

Fig. 13. The control application for the Cellavision DM1200, showing cells flagged in an automated scan.

Similarly, computer-based image analysis techniques can be applied to immunofluorescence, allowing for something almost identical to flow cytometry (appropriately named histocytometry) to occur on histologic sections of tissue.[21]

It has long been possible to create digital photosensors that can sense and collect data on spectra both below and above the limits of visible light. It is possible to capture images that include such extended data along with the visible component, and to use those data to perform extended image analysis. However, such multispectral imaging requires the use of specialized cameras, hardware, and software, which are not as readily available as the RGB-only WSI scanners that dominate the marketplace. Should multispectral imaging and histocytometry become more ubiquitous, it is possible that we will begin to move away from pure morphology as the hallmark of anatomic pathology and begin a path of convergence between the subdisciplines of anatomic and clinical pathology.[22]

By borrowing techniques from optical coherence tomography (OCT), it is possible to perform 3D reconstructions of tissue in paraffin-embedded blocks with resolutions at the tissue level, allowing for certain kinds of diagnoses (eg, complete transection of fallopian tube) to be made without the tissue ever having to be sectioned onto glass. Further study and development are required, but these techniques hold great promise.[23]

The prospect of image-based searching and pattern matching is of great interest, because such techniques would allow us to use the vast amount of data we have already stored within the pixels of existing WSI archives to further inform clinical decision support and computer-aided diagnosis. Like 3D tissue reconstruction, these techniques (including Spatial Invariant Vector Quantization) are in their infancy, and further study and development are required before they can be considered for frontline use.[24,25]

FUTURE DIRECTIONS FOR DIGITAL IMAGING IN PATHOLOGY

We are in the midst of a sea change in our discipline. As we enter the digital decade of personalized medicine, our clinicians and patients will demand greater access to integrated anatomic pathology, clinical pathology, and molecular data. We are already witnessing clinicians asking for microscopic or gross images to be attached to pathology reports or to be transmitted to their picture archiving and communication systems, and this trend will only continue. WSI will continue to advance, with slideless laboratories becoming the norm for surgical pathology, cytopathology, and hematopathology in the future.[26,27]

As we accrue both image and theranostic data, it is to hoped that the patterns embedded in these data will be unleashed to inform treatment decisions on a real-time basis by way of automated image analytical and computer-aided diagnostic algorithms. With the increasing presence of bar coding and radiofrequency identification, fine-grained tracking of pathology assets will become the rule, and our era of lost slides and misplaced cassettes will come to its well-deserved end. LISs (both of anatomic pathology and clinical pathology) will become more imaging-centric. Image analytical and computer-aided diagnostic techniques may grow so advanced that they might supplant raw morphology as the major modality of anatomic pathology diagnosis, leading to a total convergence of anatomic and clinical pathology.

Improved imaging techniques such as 3D tissue reconstruction and advanced imaging studies (eg, OCT, 4Pi microscopy, stimulated emission depletion microscopy, and other techniques) offer a tantalizing glimpse into a future in which, perhaps, our imaging technologies may become so powerful that it is no longer necessary to perform invasive biopsies to properly study a patient's disease process at the tissue or even cellular level. If this situation occurs, radiology and pathology will likely merge, creating a new diagnostic medical discipline that combines the strengths (but not the weaknesses) of its parent disciplines. We can drive such progress and take control of medicine's destiny, or we can be content to be followers or resist this disruptive technology, and eventually fade into irrelevance. The choice is ours.

REFERENCES

1. Parwani AV, Feldman M, Balis U, et al. Digital imaging. In: Pantanowitz L, Tuthill JM, Balis U, editors. Pathology informatics: theory and practice. Chicago: ASCP Press; 2012. p. 231–56.
2. Pantanowitz L, Valenstein PN, Evans AJ, et al. Review of the current state of whole slide imaging in pathology. J Pathol Inform 2011;2:36.
3. Bellina L, Missone E. Mobile cell-phones (M-phones) in telemicroscopy: increasing connectivity of isolated laboratories. Diagn Pathol 2009;4:19.
4. McLean R, Jury C, Bazeos A, et al. Application of camera phones to telehaematology. J Telemed Telecare 2009;15(7):339–43.
5. Rojo MG, Garcia GB, Mateos CP, et al. Critical comparison of 31 commercially available digital slide systems in pathology. Int J Surg Pathol 2006;14:285–305.
6. Khalbuss WE, Pantanowitz L, Parwani AV. Digital imaging in cytopathology. Patholog Res Int 2011;2011:264683.
7. Ford A. All aboard–new DICOM standard for digital images. CAP Today 2010; 25(9):94.
8. Park S, Balis U, Pantanowitz L. Computer fundamentals. In: Pantanowitz L, Tuthill JM, Balis U, editors. Pathology informatics: theory and practice. Chicago: ASCP Press; 2012. p. 11–34.
9. Sinard JH, Mattie ME. Overcoming the limitations of integrated clinical digital imaging solutions. Arch Pathol Lab Med 2005;129(9):1118–26.
10. White WL, Stavola JM. The dark side of photomicrographs in pathology reports: liability and practical concerns hidden from view. J Am Acad Dermatol 2006; 54(2):353–6.
11. Kaplan KJ, Burgess JR, Sandberg GD, et al. Use of robotic telepathology for frozen-section diagnosis: a retrospective trial of a telepathology system for intraoperative consultation. Mod Pathol 2002;15:1197–204.
12. Triola M, Hollowa W. Enhanced virtual microscopy for collaborative education. BMC Med Educ 2011;11:4.
13. Ho J, Parwani AV, Jukic DM, et al. Use of whole slide imaging on surgical pathology quality assurance design and pilot validation studies. Hum Pathol 2006;37:322–31.
14. Conway C, Dobson L, O'Grady A, et al. Virtual microscopy as an enabler of automated/quantitative assessment of protein expression in TMAs. Histochem Cell Biol 2008;130:447–63.
15. Dangott B, Parwani AV. Whole slide imaging for teleconsultation and clinical use. J Pathol Inform 2010;1:7.
16. Fine JL, Grzybicki DM, Silowash R, et al. Evaluation of whole slide image immunohistochemistry interpretation in challenging prostate needle biopsies. Hum Pathol 2008;39:564–72.
17. Gilbertson JR, Patel A, Yagi Y. Clinical slide imaging: whole slide imaging in clinical practice. In: Gu J, Oglivie RW, editors. Virtual microscopy and virtual slide in teaching, diagnosis, and research. Boca Raton (FL): Taylor & Francis; 2005. p. 225–40.

18. Pantanowitz L, Hornish M, Goulart RA. Informatics applied to cytology. Cytojournal 2008;5:16.
19. Titus K. Regulators scanning the digital scanners. CAP Today 2012;26(1):1.
20. Ceelie H, Dinkelaar RB, van Gelder W. Examination of peripheral blood films using automated microscopy; evaluation of Diffmaster Octavia and Cellavision DM96. J Clin Pathol 2007;60:72–9.
21. Al-Kofahi Y, Lassoued W, Lee W, et al. Improved automatic detection and segmentation of cell nuclei in histopathology images. IEEE Trans Biomed Eng 2010;57:841–52.
22. Angeletti C, Harvey NR, Khomitch V, et al. Detection of malignancy in cytology specimens using spectral-spatial analysis. Lab Invest 2005;85:1555–64.
23. Fine JL, Kagemann L, Wollstein G, et al. Direct scanning of pathology specimens using spectral domain optical coherence tomography: a pilot study. Ophthalmic Surg Lasers Imaging 2010;41(Suppl):S58–64.
24. Hipp JD, Cheng JY, Toner M, et al. Spatially invariant vector quantization: a pattern matching algorithm for multiple classes of image subject matter including pathology. J Pathol Inform 2011;2:13.
25. Levy BP, Hipp JD, Balis U, et al. Potential applications of digital pathology and image analysis for forensic pathology. Acad Forensic Pathol 2012;2(1):74–9.
26. Amin M, Sharma G, Parwani AV, et al. Integration of digital gross pathology images for enterprise-wide access. J Pathol Inform 2012;3:10.
27. Pantanowitz L. Digital imaging and the future of digital pathology. J Pathol Inform 2010;1:15.

Clinical Integration of Next-Generation Sequencing Technology

R.R. Gullapalli, MD, PhD[a], M. Lyons-Weiler, MS[a,c], P. Petrosko, MS[a,c],
R. Dhir, MD, MBA[a,b,c], M.J. Becich, MD, PhD[a,b,c],
W.A. LaFramboise, PhD[a,b,c],*

KEYWORDS

- Clinical pathology • Computational pathology • Genomics • Genomic sequencing
- Molecular diagnostics • Next generation sequencing • Tumor diagnostics

KEY POINTS

- There are unique requirements and limitations critical to implementation of genomic sequencing instrumentation and analysis tools in a small research laboratory or clinical environment.
- The lessons learned in the clinical integration of massively parallel sequencing technologies in genomics may be useful in the establishment of similar emerging technologies for proteomics and metabolomics.

INTRODUCTION

The development of massively parallel sequencing, also known as next-generation sequencing (NGS), has provided both basic and clinical scientists with the opportunity to carry out whole-genome sequencing in a manner previously restricted to genome centers performing large-scale sequencing projects or developing novel sequencing technologies. NGS methods have largely replaced its predecessor, Sanger dideoxynucleotide capillary sequencing, for research purposes based on greater throughput, faster readout, decreased cost per nucleotide base identification, and ease of use. Massively parallel paired-end sequencing (MPS) allows for the unprecedented global

[a] Department of Pathology, University of Pittsburgh School of Medicine, S-417 BST, 200 Lothrop Street, Pittsburgh, PA 15261, USA; [b] Department of Biomedical Informatics, University of Pittsburgh School of Medicine, 5607 Baum Boulevard, BAUM 423, Pittsburgh, PA 15206-3701, USA; [c] University of Pittsburgh Cancer Institute, Pittsburgh, PA, USA
* Corresponding author. Department of Pathology, University of Pittsburgh School of Medicine, Shadyside Hospital WG 02.11, 5230 Center Avenue, Pittsburgh, PA 15232.
E-mail address: laframboisewa@upmc.edu

Clin Lab Med 32 (2012) 585–599
http://dx.doi.org/10.1016/j.cll.2012.07.005
0272-2712/12/$ – see front matter © 2012 Elsevier Inc. All rights reserved.

assessment of interchromosomal rearrangements while simultaneously interrogating single nucleotide substitutions (also called *single nucleotide variants* [SNVs]), copy number variants (CNVs), insertions/deletions (indels), and other structural variations.[1] Discovery of novel SNVs using NGS today still requires validation via Sanger methods, because the trade-off in generating so many parallel short templates using the polymerase chain reaction (PCR) during library construction and DNA polymerase during sequencing by synthesis is loss of accuracy. NGS platforms have approximately 10-fold higher error rates (1 in 1000 bases at $20\times$ coverage) versus Sanger sequencing (1 in 10,000 bases).[1–3] However, variant call accuracy matching Sanger sequencing has been achieved at saturating coverage and 20-fold read depth per base, indicating that NGS platforms may be used as an independent discovery tool under those conditions.[3]

Next-generation platforms differ from each other predominantly in their methods of clonal amplification of short DNA fragments (50–400 bases) as a genomic library template and how these fragment libraries are subsequently sequenced through repetitive cycles to provide a nucleotide readout.[2–4] The dominant NGS whole-genome platforms are the Life Technologies SOLiD (Life Technologies Inc, Grand Island, NY), Roche 454 (Roche Diagnostics Inc, Indianapolis, IN), and Illumina systems (Illumina Inc, San Diego, CA). The SOLiD and 454 systems rely on emulsion PCR to densely decorate beads (SOLiD: 1 μm; 454: 28 μm) with monoclonal DNA templates followed by ligation sequencing or pyrosequencing, respectively, to provide a base readout. The Illumina system uses bridge PCR to amplify templates in discrete monoclonal clusters attached to the surface of a flow cell followed by reverse termination sequencing to define individual base incorporation. These platforms vary in performance characteristics and cost, and each offers advantages for different sequencing applications, such as de novo assembly versus the mapping of structural variants, but they perform comparably at saturating sequencing coverage and approach.[2–4]

The instruments, dedicated servers, and computational tools required to perform whole-genome sequencing using NGS methodology have become progressively more affordable and available through continual technological refinements since completion of the Human Genome Project. The cost of instrumentation for DNA library preparation and sequencing of whole genomes along with the computational power for data processing, transfer, storage, and analysis now fall within the price range of academic institutional core facilities ($600,000–$1 million). Smaller, less expensive instruments capable of whole exome and targeted resequencing have recently been developed for "research use only" (RUO) applications in individual research laboratories and are being avidly marketed to clinical laboratories (<$200,000). The cost of sequencing "per base" has plummeted from the estimated $2.7 billion cumulative price tag of the first genome draft sequence published in 2001 to commercial sequencing costs of $5000 for an entire genome in 2010.[2–5] At the same time, the scope of sequencing has expanded from delineation of the prototypical whole human genome to characterization of the personal genome for individualized medicine.[5,6] In particular, genomic sequencing is expected to make a preeminent contribution to diagnosis and treatment of cancer, because tumors derive from somatic DNA lesions that occur sporadically in tissues or through de novo germline changes. Carefully designed NGS studies allow characterization of multiple modalities of genomic structural alterations in cancer while providing sufficiently deep coverage to identify single-base mutations in heterogeneous specimens.[7] Translation of these discoveries into the clinical domain could subsidize a new generation of diagnostic tests. For example, important challenges regarding cancer diagnostics that can be effectively addressed using whole-genome sequencing are (1) identification of DNA biomarker regions for early diagnosis of various tumor classes, (2) delineation of genomic changes underlying the mechanisms of tumorigenesis, and (3) pretreatment specification of personal genomic alterations to validate tumor susceptibility to targeted molecular therapies.

BENCHTOP INSTRUMENTATION

Technical refinements in emulsion PCR methods, smaller flow cell size, faster microfluidics, and reduced imaging time have improved NGS speed and throughput while enabling the production of benchtop-sized sequencing instruments. The Roche 454 GS Junior, the Illumina MiSeq, and the Life Technologies Ion Torrent Personal Genome Machine (PGM) provide throughput capabilities and cost-efficiencies that support the use of these benchtop instruments in a small research laboratory environment or within a clinical diagnostic laboratory.[8] Aspects of third-generation sequencing methodology are incorporated into the Ion Torrent PGM, which interrogates single nucleotides as they are sequentially incorporated via DNA polymerase into a parallel strand complementary to the library template. The Ion Torrent PGM uses a complementary metal oxide semiconductor chip with individual wells that function as pH-sensitive pixels to directly detect the release of a hydrogen ion on nucleotide incorporation. This approach eliminates the need for chemiluminescent dyes, charged-coupled device (ccd) cameras, serial image acquisition, and a motorized stage, resulting in a faster throughput than other platforms but with shorter read lengths.[8]

Although the reduction in size, cost, and complexity of benchtop sequencers has made them more accessible, it has not improved the technical performance of their underlying NGS methodology. The Roche benchtop system still relies on pyrosequencing, and the Illumina and Ion Torrent systems perform sequencing through synthesis, thus error rates associated with those methodologies applied to short DNA fragments remain the same. The significant challenge of creating optimal template-to-bead or template-to-flow cell stoichiometry remains a critical determinant of successful sequencing in these platforms and is a major hurdle for users of these instruments. Benchtop sequencers provide the extent and depth of coverage in a single run to create a comprehensive alignment map of a bacterial genome, but require multiple runs to sequence the human exome with sufficient integrity to identify novel structural variants. However, they can readily perform high-resolution, targeted sequencing of small human genomic regions of interest in genomic domains known to be associated with diseases such as cancer. Consequently, they may prove useful for discovery research when coupled with established methods to selectively capture specific genomic target regions ranging from a few hundred bases to 500 kilobases (kb) using primer-driven amplification, hybridization-based capture, or restriction digest isolation (Agilent, Inc, Carlsbad, CA; Roche Nimblegen, Inc, Madison, WI; Life Technologies, Inc).[9]

The falling cost of genomic sequencing has driven rapid growth of NGS use in RUO applications involving the sequencing of DNA from fresh-frozen and formalin-fixed paraffin-embedded (FFPE) specimens. Although peculiarities exist that are specific to FFPE preparations, studies have shown critical common sources of errors associated with implementing whole-genome sequencing platforms, which should be considered when using benchtop versions of these instruments. However, the short reads and depth of coverage associated with NGS systems yield high-fidelity single-base interrogation of FFPE samples compared with microarray and PCR assays.

Extrinsic or preanalytic variables that can affect sequence accuracy and integrity at the level of sample acquisition and processing include specimen cellular heterogeneity, DNA extraction method, reagent batch effects, protocol drift, nucleotide or barcode cross-contamination, personnel training, and study site. Many of these factors can be balanced through randomizing the order of sample processing, procuring large reagent lots, altering the position of DNA samples within plates, and including interbatch positive and negative sequencing controls. The sequencing platforms and instrumentation are themselves an intrinsic source of variability affecting technical reproducibility, accuracy, error rates, and the specificity and sensitivity to detect genomic structural changes down to the level of mutant alleles. The performance of NGS methods and instruments should be routinely validated against a laboratory DNA standard, such as a Hap Map cell line without somatic variants and a tumor cell line with stable structural changes and mutations. An average depth of sequence coverage of $50\times$ or greater is adequate for validating these homogeneous samples. However, for clinical samples comprising tumor cells that are contained within an admixture of heterogeneous cells (eg, stroma, infiltrating immune cells, capillary endothelial cells), a much deeper coverage ($100\times$–$1000\times$) is generally required. Despite precise error control and calibration standards, concern persists as to whether NGS platforms independently provide the confidence levels required for using previously uncharacterized novel individual variant calls in clinical samples for patient diagnostic applications.

The value that NGS technology could bring to clinical laboratory diagnostic services is accentuated by several recent genetic developments. First, next-generation genomic sequencing was critical to the characterization of genetic disorders over the past decade, with nearly 3000 single-gene Mendelian disorders identified by 2011.[10] Second, increased numbers of small molecule–targeted cancer therapies have been introduced over the past decade that require a sequence-based companion diagnostic test (eg, the drug PLX-4032 targets papillary thyroid cancers and metastatic malignant melanoma that feature the V600E mutation of the *BRAF* gene).[11] As the number of these therapeutic products increases, the demand for sequencing solid tumors and hematologic malignancies will commensurately increase. Third, multi-gene cancer biomarker panels have emerged that provide diagnostic information in demand by both patients and physicians. For example, Oncotype DX, PAM50, and MammaPrint are separate gene expression assays that supply information on the risk of breast cancer recurrence and help inform therapy choices through evaluation of 21, 50, and 70 genes, respectively.[12,13] The role of the clinical diagnostic laboratory in generating genomic information associated with these developments is not clear. However, it is certain that increased demand for detailed patient genomic information for diagnosis and treatment cannot be met by scaling up traditional Sanger sequencing, pyrosequencing, or PCR methods, whereas NGS can acutely meet the challenge.

For benchtop sequencing platforms to be effective in hospital clinical laboratories for diagnostic purposes, they must provide rapid sample throughput and turnaround times (minutes to hours), use standardized protocols including positive and negative technical controls, and obtain reimbursement within current acceptable guidelines (hundreds to thousands of dollars). The turnaround time promoted for benchtop sequencing instruments attempts to satisfy these clinical laboratory requirements, particularly with the use of DNA barcoding adapters that allow multiple samples to be evaluated simultaneously. The significant labor and costs of capturing, amplifying, and preparing templates for targeted sequencing, and the time and resources required to perform the data analysis are currently within the time frame and price point for clinical laboratories using the fastest benchtop NGS systems.

Protocols for NGS are marketed as semiautomated and easy to use. In the authors' experience, commercial sequencing protocols are still undergoing routine revision, lack important quality assurance and quality control checkpoints, and are subject to version drift. Furthermore, the highest acuity for identifying critical genomic alterations in tumor samples is through direct comparison with DNA obtained from a normal sample, preferably blood. The addition of a matched normal reference doubles the cost, required reagents, and work effort. Consequently, the development, validation, and accreditation of sequencing tests to supplant current accredited stand-alone assays are unlikely. A more probable scenario for clinical laboratory sequencing is implementation of new diagnostic tests revealed through NGS on whole-genome platforms but translated into targeted assays for benchtop instruments. These tests will evaluate larger genomic domains at high resolution to provide physicians with knowledge that is currently unattainable through Sanger sequencing or quantitative PCR, such as the presence of unexpected sequence structural abnormalities, somatic base pairs and indels, balanced and unbalanced somatic rearrangements, and gene copy number information, including homozygous and heterozygous deletions associated with specific diseases.

ENTERPRISE SEQUENCING

The advent of massively parallel sequencing has enabled an intense effort at the enterprise level to characterize various normal and tumor genomes through drawing on the infrastructure and expertise developed during the Human Genome Project. Multiple large-scale sequencing projects are underway in an effort to accumulate genomic data from patients with cancer in centralized databases and concurrently develop analytic tools for interrogating these data. Examples in cancer genomics include The Cancer Genome Atlas (National Cancer Institute and National Human Genome Research Institute [NHGRI]), the Cancer Genome Project (Wellcome Trust Sanger Institute), and the International Cancer Genome Consortium (Ontario Institute for Cancer Research).[14,15] Individual institutions, such as the Genome Institute at Washington University in St. Louis, have developed independent programs, such as the Pediatric Cancer Genome Project building on expertise developed during the Human Genome Project. Companies providing commercial targeted and whole-genome services are also rapidly proliferating as service providers and data repositories (**Table 1**). These programs will no doubt continue to multiply based on the assumption that accumulation of DNA sequence and detailed clinical data will achieve a critical mass when the appropriate analysis of a comprehensive sequence repository will answer pertinent scientific and clinical questions, such as identifying driver mutations as therapeutic targets and predicting patient response to therapy.

NGS DATA ANALYSIS

Most commercial NGS platforms generate light (fluorescence) as the underlying raw signal output when the genomic template is interrogated with serial images accumulating until they are converted to a base readout. Once the base coding is obtained for the templates, it requires a computationally intensive process to map these sequence fragments in register with an established reference sequence as opposed to the complex task of de novo assembly. The current standard is the latest build of the human genome provided by the Genome Reference Consortium.[15]

A typical supercomputing DNA alignment solution uses multiple parallel processing nodes to assemble different genomic components of the data. The head node subsequently aggregates these data to provide a final mapped genomic sequence. The computer processing time required for mapping depends on the extent of the mapped genome (genome, exome, or target region) and the redundancy of coverage. A single

Table 1
Select vendors of commercial genomics and data storage services as of June 2012

Service	Vendor	Web site	Remarks
Whole Genome Sequencing (WGS)	Complete Genomics	www.completegenomics.com	Using various NGS technologies, these vendors provide WGS services within several weeks to months of sample submission
	Seqwright	www.seqwright.com	The data are provided in a raw format without any interpretation of the variants
Whole Exome Sequencing (WES)	Ambry Genetics	www.ambrygen.com	The focus of WES services is to sequence the protein (± microRNA) coding part of the genome, including their splice sites
	Baylor College of Medicine	www.bcm.edu	The whole exome is "captured" by using specially designed bait probes
	Emory University	http://genetics.emory.edu	
Genomic data storage providers	Amazon Web services	http://aws.amazon.com	Commercial storage and computing power in the "cloud"
	Microsoft cloud services	www.windowsazure.com	Prices are highly competitive with enormous computing power at one's fingertips
	Rackspace	www.rackspace.com	However, issues related to patient privacy and HIPAA compliance remain
			Amazon has taken initial steps to ensure compliance with Health Insurance Portability and Accountability Act
			Data transfer of the huge WES and WGS data files over the Internet is a significant problem
Genome/exome interpretation software/ providers	Personalis	www.personalis.com	The goal of commercial companies in the data interpretation space is to interpret the raw sequence data for a fee
	Omicia	www.omicia.com	The data may be generated in-house or from an external source
	Knome	www.knome.com	Most of the bioinformatics tools are developed on a proprietary basis
	Cypher Genomics	http://cyphergenomics.com	Information related to pathway analysis, sequence variants, and data-querying services are provided
	SvBio	www.svbio.com	Most of these companies are in the incubator stage
	Genomatix	www.genomatix.de	
	Omixon	www.omixon.com	

This list is not exhaustive and is intended for initial guidance only.

base of the human haploid genome occupies roughly 2.5 bytes in the FASTQ format. Mapping the 3.1-gigabase whole human genome at 30× coverage generates 2.5 × 3.1 × 30× or approximately 230 gigabases of raw base calls requiring hours of parallel processing. The alignment process is complicated by the fact that the fragment data comprises inherently self-similar FASTQ text lines. NGS technology can currently be implemented in a medium-sized facility (eg, an academic medical center), because computer capabilities have increased in speed and decreased in cost. A potential schematic of the NGS workflow is shown in **Fig. 1**.

The goal of clinical NGS for cancer diagnostics is the identification of pertinent point mutations and larger structural variations, such as translocations, rearrangements, inversions, deletions, and amplifications in tumor samples compared with the normal genome. Currently an array of free and commercially available software are available for NGS data analysis. The workflow includes 3 major steps.

Step 1: Alignment and Assembly

Multiple free mapping software tools are available, including MAQ,[16] BWA,[17] Bowtie,[18] SOAP,[19] ZOOM,[20] SHRiMP,[21] and Novoalign.[22] Illumina and SOLiD also provide their own alignment software. Commercial third-party software vendors such as CLC Genomics also provide mapping programs. Disadvantages of free open source software are the lack of documentation and a reliance on Unix and its command-line

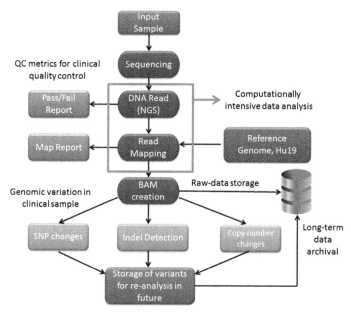

Fig. 1. Prototypical workflow in a clinical next generation sequencing laboratory. The entire workflow process occurs under the auspices of a Clinical Laboratory Improvement Amendments–certified laboratory (CLIA) for clinical diagnostic application. An important distinction of the workflow process in the clinical laboratory relative to a research environment is enforcement of strict process and quality metrics. Currently, a national standard for quality assurance in an NGS laboratory remains to be defined. BAM, Binary Alignment Map; SNP, Single Nucleotide Polymorphism; Indel, Insertions-Deletions; Hu19, human genome reference assembly.

environment. However, open source software based on the Burrows-Wheeler transformation (BWT) algorithm remains significantly faster than commercial solutions for mapping and alignment. Software based on the BWT algorithm can map a human genome in hours instead of days, as required by other software tools such as MAQ[16] and Novoalign.[22] Commercial vendors provide access to proprietary mapping algorithms but at a substantial cost for mid-level academic institutions. Software for de novo assembly of cancer genomes, such as Velvet,[23,24] EULER-SR,[25] EDENA,[26] QSR,[27] and AbYSS,[28] is a powerful tool for detecting unique rearrangements and chromosomal breakpoints in a tumor sample, albeit through a slower method than mapping against the reference genome.

Step 2: Variant Detection

Once alignment is completed, downstream bioinformatics analysis is performed to detect structural genomic alterations relevant to the clinical diagnosis.

1. Single-nucleotide polymorphisms (SNPs) and point mutations: molecular diagnostic assays for cancer have focused on discovery of mutations in tumor-related genes or small panels of these genes. For example, certain mutations in the epidermal growth factor receptor (EGFR) gene are associated with favorable responses in lung cancers treated with gefitinib compared with lung cancers with wild-type EGFR.[29] An impediment to finding these somatic mutations in cancer is specimen cellular heterogeneity. Recent studies indicate that there is a 5% probability of detecting a mutation in 25% of tumor cells sequenced at 30- to 40-fold coverage.[30] Laser capture microdissection to obtain DNA from a population highly enriched for cancer cells can reduce the cellular variability of the specimen. A variety of software tools are available for detecting single nucleotide variants based on different statistical models of base-calling, including SNVmix,[31] VarScan,[32] and SomaticSniper.[33] Open source tools, such as SAMtools,[34] use Bayesian detection to identify somatic SNP variants.

2. Structural changes in the cancer genome: cancer genomes are highly unstable, containing diverse chromosomal abnormalities such as large genomic insertions and deletions. Although karyotyping is the standard method to identify chromosomal abnormalities, it cannot identify structural abnormalities smaller than approximately 5 megabases. SNP and oligonucleotide microarrays have revolutionized the field of cytogenetics, providing high-resolution (~1 kb) to identify copy number variants and copy neutral loss of heterozygosity. NGS technologies also identify structural variations in the genome, although typical alignment tools cannot identify more than a few nucleotide mismatches. Specialized software for analyzing indels from paired-end reads, such as Pindel,[35] identify structural variants by defining the flanking regions of the read data while the GATK indel genotyper[36] uses heuristic cutoffs for indel calling. Nevertheless, delineation of large amplifications and deletions in cancer chromosomes remains a formidable challenge. Algorithms to identify large variations include the circular binary segmentation algorithm of arrays[37] and the SegSeq algorithm, which uses a merging procedure to join localized SNP changes with whole chromosome changes to compare tumor and normal samples.[38] Several programs are available to identify large-scale structural variations in the genome, such as BreakDancer.[39] Although NGS technology has revealed variations in lung cancer, melanomas, and breast cancer at the single nucleotide level,[7,40–43] significant hurdles remain in addressing changes at the chromosomal level.

Step 3: Beyond Genome Sequencing

NGS platforms offer the versatility to perform transcriptomic profiling, chromatin immunoprecipitation, small RNA sequencing, and epigenomic studies. Transcriptomics via NGS can probe alternate splicing, the process through which multiple RNA isoforms arise from a single gene. These isoforms contribute to cell type specificity and may play a role in specification of cancerous cells. Identification of novel splicing variants is important for understanding biologic specificity in the context of normal and abnormal cellular function. Software tools such as TOPHAT[44] facilitate de novo discovery of splicing variants.

RNA discovery

The role of small RNAs (18–35 base pairs) in the regulation of gene expression and translation of mRNAs has been recognized recently. NGS methods can perform deep sequencing of small RNA species for discovery and analysis. Platforms such as Illumina and SOLiD have a specific advantage in small RNA discovery because of the short reads they generate. Many small RNA databases and bioinformatics tools are available, such as MirCat[45] and mirDeep,[46,47] that can facilitate identification and discovery of small RNAs.

Epigenomic discovery

Epigenomics refers to chemical modifications (eg, methylation) of DNA and RNA and the impact on gene expression. Traditional methods of assessing gene methylation rely on bisulfite conversion of unmethylated cytosines to uracil for identification using sequencing methods or restriction endonuclease analysis. One pitfall associated with this approach is the labor-intensive methodology required to identify epigenetic changes on an individual gene basis. In contrast, NGS technologies can interrogate broad changes in DNA methylation patterns across the entire genome, simultaneously capturing epigenetic information from multiple genes while providing information regarding normal or tumor tissue methylation status.

SCIENTIFIC CHALLENGES FOR THE IMPLEMENTATION OF NGS

The acuity of cancer-related sequencing studies is enhanced by differential comparison of patient tumor genomic sequences with matched normal reference sequences, such as a paired blood sample. However, routine assembly and comparison of each of these paired samples is dependent on the existence of an accurate representation of the reference human normal genome, including its intrinsic variability encompassing benign structural modifications and polymorphisms. A database comprising normal whole-genome sequences is being compiled through concomitant large parallel sequencing projects, including the 1000 Genomes Project (NHGRI; an extension of the International HapMap Project), the Genome Reference Consortium (Wellcome Trust, Genome Institute at Washington University, European Molecular Biology Laboratory, National Center for Biotechnology Information) and the Personal Genome Project (Harvard University).[48–50] The initial reference genome was constructed de novo with DNA from a small number of anonymous subjects, with the bulk of the clones (~60%) from a single male donor. The current iteration of the reference genome (Genome Reference Consortium 37 or HG Build19) is estimated to be 99.99% accurate, containing 2.95 billion bases and 210 gaps.[49] Sequencing of personal genomes has established diversity as high as 3% among individuals, and personal sequences can differ from the reference genome in hundreds of thousands of bases.[51,52] These estimates will likely change drastically with accumulating numbers of personal genome sequences. Thus, the current reference genome represents only a small sampling of human genetic variation and contains thousands of both common and rare risk alleles that remain to be defined.

It is also important to consider relevant limitations learned from previous public and private enterprise computing efforts regarding population-based genomics. For example, the HapMap Project and deCODE Genetics were initiated more than a decade ago as public and private enterprises with the goal of exhaustively mapping population-based genetic diversity on a worldwide basis or within the restricted population of the Icelandic Health Sector.[53] The hypothesis underlying these efforts was that disease- and treatment-related variants would emerge as these databases and analytic tools succeeded in precisely characterizing normal specimens and delineating differences specific to diseased samples.

Although significant discoveries continue to be made from these efforts, several important issues have emerged pertinent to cancer initiatives. First, the classification of "normal" specimens is challenging, because they may either originate from truly disease-free subjects or derive from asymptomatic patients harboring undiagnosed disease. Second, classification of a tumor specimen may vary. Some tumors are difficult to classify, whereas other definitive tumor types have undergone subsequent phenotype reclassification, further confounding their annotation and interrogation because of the persistence of legacy classifications. Third, multisite genomic data generation produces differences in data fidelity, variability, precision, and accuracy associated with the use of different methodologies, instruments, reagent lots, experimental batches, and personnel. Because of the increased noise-to-signal ratio at the consortium level, many frustrated investigators have created their own in-house reference databases to obviate issues encountered at the enterprise level. This experience from the previous decade is equally relevant today as genomic sequencing databases are being generated.

INSTITUTIONAL CHALLENGES FOR THE IMPLEMENTATION OF NGS

Bioinformatics is currently the single largest bottleneck to implementation of NGS in clinical practice. A general guideline is that each dollar spent on sequencing hardware will require an equal investment in informatics.[54] Smaller laboratories cannot absorb these costs, even with the availability of open source software.[55] Several critical considerations must be addressed in developing an NGS bioinformatics facility. NGS hardware implementation requires substantial investment in infrastructure. Alternatively, this task can be outsourced to a commercial third-party provider. However, in-house sequencing and analysis enables important control of sample substrate, library creation, sequence generation, and data processing. This ownership is critical for clinical diagnostic sequencing, wherein process and quality control are of utmost priority. As NGS technology is applied to clinical problems, standardizing quality metrics for acquisition of data is critical. These metrics include standards for calibration, validation, and comparison among platforms; data reliability, robustness, and reproducibility; and quality of assemblers. Guidelines for standardization of NGS protocols will need to be developed, such as occurred in the microarray quality control (MAQC)[56] and sequencing quality control (SEQC, or MAQC-III) projects (http://www.fda.gov/MicroArrayQC/), particularly as laboratory-developed tests (LDT) emerge outside the federal regulatory domain.

Most academic centers have existing centralized computing resources that can be leveraged for in-house NGS analysis by upgrading to high-performance computer clusters. However, the need for advanced network infrastructure is a formidable barrier to implementing NGS in a research or clinical setting. The typical academic network architecture comprises 100-MB shared Ethernet services or a lower bandwidth wide-area network (WAN) infrastructure. Because NGS data sets are hundreds of gigabytes per run, efficient data transfer requires 10-gigabit network connectivity with gigabit cabling between locations, including high-speed network switching and network cards on devices that serve the network. Consequently, most academic and many commercial service providers transport their data via portable hard drives and other mobile transfer solutions, including transfer from sequencer to server. Advantages of an in-house network for data transfer and analysis include scheduled maintenance, professional backup facilities, direct security oversight, and dedicated and/or shared nodes for research. **Fig. 1** depicts a routine bioinformatics workflow required for analysis of NGS data.

The amount of data generated by the sequencing of a single genome comprises hundreds of gigabytes of base calls and quality scores. Multiple runs rapidly accumulate in the terabyte range, and a clinical NGS center could produce terabytes to a petabyte of data in a year. Data management on this scale requires well-defined policies and standards, although few exist. Furthermore, no industry-wide standardization exists for data output from NGS platforms, with the most commonly accepted forms comprising SAM (Sequence Alignment/Map) and BAM (Binary Alignment Map) formats.[34] BAM files store the data in a compressed, indexed, binary data file format (binary text–based format) for efficient storage. NGS data can be stored either (1) locally on the instrument, (2) at an institutional storage facility, or (3) using a commercial cloud storage solution. NGS data is more convenient to store institutionally or commercially rather than locally. Cloud computing is an especially promising data storage solution; however, privacy and security must be ensured to meet rigid Health Insurance Portability and Accountability Act (HIPAA) requirements.

Online computer clusters have become commercially available for public on-demand access in the form of cloud computing solutions. Amazon, Google, and Microsoft have created centralized supercomputing facilities through virtualization of software, a process whereby a user can access an image of the operating system (Linux or Windows) residing on the server of the company hosting the cloud. This interface image is indistinguishable from an ordinary desktop interface. The difference is that the virtual operating system is hosted on a remote server (**Fig. 2**).

The advantage of a cloud solution is access to supercomputing power without installation and maintenance of expensive hardware. Fees for cloud services are

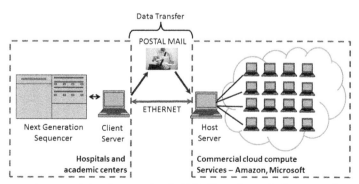

Fig. 2. Prospective use of cloud computing in NGS. The schematic illustrates the transfer of data from a sequencing instrument to a commercial cloud vendor service through the Internet or using regular postal mail. Subsequent analysis may be performed remotely from the sequencing laboratory domain.

currently affordable for an average user, with pay-as-you-go pricing. Private vendors, such as Amazon S3 (Simple Storage Service), also provide long-term storage of datasets through networked storage facilities, a critically important issue given the scale of NGS datasets. Disadvantages with cloud services include satisfaction of HIPAA compliance and security of data transfer over a vulnerable Internet network. Another critical variable is the insurance policy regarding long-term storage and protection of clinical data in a commercial environment in which ownership is subject to change, merger, or acquisition.

TRAINING AND IMPLEMENTATION OF NGS IN THE CLINICAL WORKPLACE

Analysis of NGS data requires multidisciplinary teams of clinical and biomedical/pathology informaticians, computational biologists, molecular pathologists, programmers, statisticians, biologists, and clinicians. Consequently, substantial institutional support for resources and personnel is needed for clinical implementation of NGS technology. Furthermore, physicians will have to be trained to interpret vast and comprehensive molecular data sets. Currently, there are approximately 1000 medical geneticists and 3000 genetic counselors in the United States. These numbers are grossly inadequate to deal with the explosive growth of genomics testing. One solution is to form strategic collaborations between disciplines. For example, more than 17,000 pathologists in the United States have broad education in anatomic pathology and laboratory medicine who could undergo further trained to integrate large data sets with clinical findings.[57] Specifically, a need exists to create a subspecialty of "computational pathology" to train pathologists to manage and interpret high-throughput biologic data, including that derived from genomic, proteomic, and metabolomics analysis.

SUMMARY

The development of massively parallel sequencing methods has expanded genomic sequencing from delineating the prototypical reference human genome to characterization of the individual patient genome as the building block of personalized medicine. The accessibility of this technology has produced important results from the small research laboratory to enterprise-level analysis regarding genomic changes associated with cancer. Benchtop systems incorporating NGS technology have been recently released and are being marketed to the clinical laboratory to meet the demand for personalized medicine applications. To achieve long-term success in the clinical domain, critical requirements include the development of versatile, robust, and affordable instrument platforms; the development of user-friendly bioinformatics tools and support; and evolution of a workforce with pertinent knowledge of molecular biology and genomics. If successful, these systems will provide an incomparable level of diagnostic insight for patients as novel genomic biomarkers and structural changes are identified for application to the clinical domain.

REFERENCES

1. Campbell PJ, Stephens PJ, Pleasance ED, et al. Identification of somatically acquired rearrangements in cancer using genome-wide massively parallel paired-end sequencing. Nat Genet 2008;40(6):722–9.
2. Shendure J, Ji H. Next-generation DNA sequencing. Nat Biotechnol 2008;26(10): 1135–45.

3. Harismendy O, Ng PC, Strausberg RL, et al. Evaluation of next generation sequencing platforms for population targeted sequencing studies. Genome Biol 2009;10(3):R32.
4. Metzker ML. Sequencing technologies - the next generation. Nat Rev Genet 2010;11(1):31–46.
5. Ross JS, Cronin M. Whole cancer genome sequencing by next-generation methods. Am J Clin Pathol 2011;136(4):527–39.
6. West M, Ginsburg GS, Huang AT, et al. Embracing the complexity of genomic data for personalized medicine. Genome Res 2006;16(5):559–66.
7. Shah SP, Morin RD, Khattra J, et al. Mutational evolution in a lobular breast tumour profiled at single nucleotide resolution. Nature 2009;461(7265):809–13.
8. Loman NJ, Misra RV, Dallman TJ, et al. Performance comparison of bench top high-throughput sequencing platforms. Nat Biotechnol 2012;30:434–9.
9. Horn S. Target enrichment via DNA hybridization capture. Methods Mol Biol 2012; 840:177–88.
10. Feero WG, Guttmacher AE, Collins FS. Genomic medicine–an updated primer. N Engl J Med 2010;362(21):2001–11.
11. Lee JT, Li L, Brafford PA, et al. PLX4032, a potent inhibitor of the B-Raf V600E oncogene, selectively inhibits V600E-positive melanomas. Pigment Cell Melanoma Res 2010;23(6):820–7.
12. Kelly CM, Bernard PS, Krishnamurthy S, et al. Agreement in risk prediction between the 21-gene recurrence score assay (Oncotype DX(R)) and the PAM50 breast cancer intrinsic Classifier™ in early-stage estrogen receptor-positive breast cancer. Oncologist 2012;17(4):492–8.
13. van de Vijver MJ, He YD, van't Veer LJ, et al. A gene-expression signature as a predictor of survival in breast cancer. N Engl J Med 2002;347(25):1999–2009.
14. Collins FS, Barker AD. Mapping the cancer genome. Pinpointing the genes involved in cancer will help chart a new course across the complex landscape of human malignancies. Sci Am 2007;296(3):50–7.
15. International Cancer Genome Consortium. International network of cancer genome projects. Nature 2010;464(7291):993–8.
16. Li H, Ruan J, Durbin R. Mapping short DNA sequencing reads and calling variants using mapping quality scores. Genome Res 2008;18(11):1851–8.
17. Lippert RA, Mobarry CM, Walenz BP. A space-efficient construction of the Burrows-Wheeler transform for genomic data [review]. J Comput Biol 2005;12(7):943–51.
18. Pop M, Salzberg SL. Bioinformatics challenges of new sequencing technology [review]. Trends Genet 2008;24(3):142–9.
19. Li R, Li Y, Kristiansen K, et al. SOAP: short oligonucleotide alignment program. Bioinformatics 2008;24(5):713–4.
20. Lin H, Zhang Z, Zhang MQ, et al. ZOOM! Zillions of oligos mapped. Bioinformatics 2008;24(21):2431–7.
21. Rumble SM, Lacroute P, Dalca AV, et al. SHRiMP: accurate mapping of short color-space reads. PLoS Comput Biol 2009;5(5):e1000386.
22. Bao S, Jiang R, Kwan W, et al. Evaluation of next-generation sequencing software in mapping and assembly. J Hum Genet 2011;56(6):406–14.
23. Zerbino DR, Birney E. Velvet: algorithms for de novo short read assembly using de Bruijn graphs. Genome Res 2008;18(5):821–9.
24. Zerbino DR. Using the Velvet de novo assembler for short-read sequencing technologies. Curr Protoc Bioinformatics 2010;11(11):5.
25. Chaisson MJ, Pevzner PA. Short read fragment assembly of bacterial genomes. Genome Res 2008;18(2):324–30.

26. Hernandez D, François P, Farinelli L, et al. De novo bacterial genome sequencing: millions of very short reads assembled on a desktop computer. Genome Res 2008;18(5):802–9.
27. Bryant DW Jr, Wong WK, Mockler TC. QSRA: a quality-value guided de novo short read assembler. BMC Bioinformatics 2009;10:69.
28. Simpson JT, Wong K, Jackman SD, et al. ABySS: a parallel assembler for short read sequence data. Genome Res 2009;19(6):1117–23.
29. Paez JG, Jänne PA, Lee JC, et al. EGFR mutations in lung cancer: correlation with clinical response to gefitinib therapy. Science 2004;304(5676):1497–500.
30. Nik-Zainal S, Van Loo P, Wedge DC, et al, Breast Cancer Working Group of the International Cancer Genome Consortium. The life history of 21 breast cancers. Cell 2012;149(5):994–1007.
31. Goya R, Sun MG, Morin RD, et al. SNVMix: predicting single nucleotide variants from next-generation sequencing of tumors. Bioinformatics 2010;26(6):730–6.
32. Koboldt DC, Zhang Q, Larson DE, et al. VarScan 2: somatic mutation and copy number alteration discovery in cancer by exome sequencing. Genome Res 2012;22(3):568–76.
33. Larson DE, Harris CC, Chen K, et al. SomaticSniper: identification of somatic point mutations in whole genome sequencing data. Bioinformatics 2012;28(3):311–7.
34. Li H, Handsaker B, Wysoker A, et al, 1000 Genome Project Data Processing Subgroup. The Sequence Alignment/Map format and SAMtools. Bioinformatics 2009;25(16):2078–9.
35. Ye K, Schulz MH, Long Q, et al. Pindel: a pattern growth approach to detect break points of large deletions and medium sized insertions from paired-end short reads. Bioinformatics 2009;25(21):2865–71.
36. DePristo MA, Banks E, Poplin R, et al. A framework for variation discovery and genotyping using next-generation DNA sequencing data. Nat Genet 2011;43(5):491–8.
37. Campbell PJ, Yachida S, Mudie LJ, et al. The patterns and dynamics of genomic instability in metastatic pancreatic cancer. Nature 2010;467(7319):1109–13.
38. Chiang DY, Getz G, Jaffe DB, et al. High-resolution mapping of copy-number alterations with massively parallel sequencing. Nat Methods 2009;6(1):99–103.
39. Chen K, Wallis JW, McLellan MD, et al. BreakDancer: an algorithm for high-resolution mapping of genomic structural variation. Nat Methods 2009;6(9):677–81.
40. Stransky N, Egloff AM, Tward AD, et al. The mutational landscape of head and neck squamous cell carcinoma. Science 2011;333(6046):1157–60.
41. Verhaak RG, Hoadley KA, Purdom E, et al, Cancer Genome Atlas Research Network. Integrated genomic analysis identifies clinically relevant subtypes of glioblastoma characterized by abnormalities in PDGFRA, IDH1, EGFR, and NF1. Cancer Cell 2010;17(1):98–110.
42. Berger MF, Levin JZ, Vijayendran K, et al. Integrative analysis of the melanoma transcriptome. Genome Res 2010;20(4):413–27.
43. Weir BA, Woo MS, Getz G, et al. Characterizing the cancer genome in lung adenocarcinoma. Nature 2007;450(7171):893–8.
44. Trapnell C, Pachter L, Salzberg SL. TopHat: discovering splice junctions with RNA-Seq. Bioinformatics 2009;25(9):1105–11.
45. Moxon S, Schwach F, Dalmay T, et al. A toolkit for analysing large-scale plant small RNA datasets. Bioinformatics 2008;24(19):2252–3.

46. Friedländer MR, Chen W, Adamidi C, et al. Discovering microRNAs from deep sequencing data using miRDeep. Nat Biotechnol 2008;26(4):407–15.
47. Yang X, Li L. miRDeep-P: a computational tool for analyzing the microRNA transcriptome in plants. Bioinformatics 2011;27(18):2614–5.
48. 1000 Genomes Project Consortium. A map of human genome variation from population-scale sequencing. Nature 2010;467(7319):1061–73.
49. International Human Genome Sequencing Consortium. Finishing the euchromatic sequence of the human genome. Nature 2004;431(7011):931–45.
50. Personal Genome Project. Available at: http://www.personalgenomes.org. Accessed May 21, 2012.
51. Venter JC. Multiple personal genomes await. Nature 2010;464(7289):676–7.
52. International HapMap 3 Consortium. Integrating common and rare genetic variation in diverse human populations. Nature 2010;467(7311):52–8.
53. Gulcher J, Stefansson K. Population genomics: laying the groundwork for genetic disease modeling and targeting. Clin Chem Lab Med 1998;36(8):523–7.
54. Perkel JM. Sequence analysis 101: a newbie's guide to crunching next-generation sequencing data. Scientist 2011;25:60.
55. Maxmen A. Harnessing the cloud. Scientist 2010;24:71.
56. Patterson TA, Lobenhofer EK, Fulmer-Smentek SB, et al. Performance comparison of one-color and two-color platforms within the MicroArray Quality Control (MAQC) project. Nat Biotechnol 2006;24(9):1140–50.
57. Haspel RL, Arnaout R, Briere L, et al. A call to action: training pathology residents in genomics and personalized medicine. Am J Clin Pathol 2010;133(6):832–4.

Workflow Organization in Pathology

Seung Park, MD*, Liron Pantanowitz, MD,
Anil Vasdev Parwani, MD, PhD, Alan Wells, MD, Zoltán N. Oltvai, MD

KEYWORDS

- Clinical pathology • Anatomic pathology • Genomics • Molecular diagnostics
- Modeling • Workflow organization

KEY POINTS

- An understanding of workflow science is critical for the practicing pathologist because it enables him or her to become an agent of positive change at an institutional level.
- Workflows can be sorted into three models: preindustrial, industrial, and postindustrial. Each workflow model has its advantages and disadvantages.
- The pathology workflow features a blend of preindustrial and industrial elements; the clinical pathology workflow currently features far more automation than the anatomic pathology workflow.
- Though laboratory information systems provide the electronic backbone on which the modern pathology department provides its services, these systems are often rigid and not interoperable.
- The lessons of the Toyota Production System are especially relevant to pathology because the pathology workflow arguably shares more similarities with a manufacturing workflow than any other workflow in medicine.

INTRODUCTION

Workflow organization in the pathology laboratory is not a topic that is well-understood, sometimes even by those who claim to be experts in the field. This largely because any given real-world production process is usually only observed one component at a time by stakeholders who are primarily concerned with that component (often in isolation). In surgical pathology, for instance, the histotechnologist, the slide custodian, and the pathologist all engage in the tracking of a very specific set of assets (ie, glass slides), yet their reasons for doing so may be quite different. As a result, their conclusions about the production process in which they operate and,

The authors have no relationships (financial, commercial, or otherwise) to disclose.
Department of Pathology, University of Pittsburgh Medical Center, UPMC Shadyside Hospital Suite 201, 5150 Centre Avenue, Pittsburgh, PA 15232, USA
* Corresponding author.
E-mail address: parks3@upmc.edu

Clin Lab Med 32 (2012) 601–622
http://dx.doi.org/10.1016/j.cll.2012.07.008
0272-2712/12/$ – see front matter © 2012 Elsevier Inc. All rights reserved.

labmed.theclinics.com

perhaps more importantly, their reactions to the errors that arise within that system can be widely divergent.

Historically, in organizing its workflow, medicine has chosen to follow the lead of the manufacturing industry, deriving most of its quality control measures from practices that happened to be in vogue in the manufacturing sector at the time. A search (done June 2012) of PubMed using the search terms "quality management" and "laboratory" yielded 845 articles from 1966 to the present that focuses Total Quality Management to Six Sigma to Lean production on production management paradigms from. Although many (if not all) of these articles describe successful implementation of one production management paradigm or another in the health care sector, it is revealing that (1) health care providers still routinely encounter the same kinds of medical error that these production management paradigms are purported to solve, (2) the overarching culture of medicine has arguably remained largely unchanged, and (3) the mastercrafter-apprentice model of physician training has (at least for now) remained dominant. All of these observations have far-reaching implications that are discussed below.

Medicine is becoming more data-centric and patient-centric every passing day (ie, personalized medicine). As representatives of the medical discipline that generates and warehouses most of the average medical record's structured data, pathologists have the opportunity to be the drivers of optimal workflow organization in a radically changing practice environment. To this end, however, all pathologists should have a basic understanding of the principles of workflow organization and production management and their modes of implementation. It is the authors' hope that this article will provide such a foundation and inspire our colleagues to be champions of relentless quality improvement.

HISTORICAL OVERVIEW

The history of workflow organization can be divided into three distinct phases: preindustrial, industrial, and postindustrial.

Preindustrial Workflow

The preindustrial workflow is characterized by a high concentration of knowledge and skill in the hands of individual craftspeople who attain their position through time-intensive, idiosyncratic training programs (ie, apprentice to journeyman to master), usually under the direction of one master. Before the development and popularization of assembly line-style production methods in the mid-nineteenth to early twentieth century, this was the dominant workflow model in every industry in the world. In certain disciplines (notably, medicine) this remains the dominant model for training and professional licensure (ie, the medical student to resident to fellow to attending progression) even today.

In the preindustrial workflow, individual talent and attention to detail are major determinants of the resultant product. In addition, each master has a highly-customized workflow that may bear only superficial resemblance to the workflow of his or her peers. Finally, a master is also limited by the tools and raw materials he or she has on hand. It should, therefore, come as no surprise that the preindustrial workflow exhibits relatively high variability in the quality of and between masters. The preindustrial workflow's focus on individual craftspersons leads to a curious phenomenon in which individual masters can build reputations that far overshadow the objective quality of their works. The world of classical music provides us with a fascinating example: violins by Antonio Stradivari and Giuseppe Guarneri (del Gesù) are widely considered superior to all others even though repeated double-blind studies show that even highly-regarded professional violinists cannot tell the difference between a Stradivarius, a Guarneri del Gesù, and a well-crafted violin by a modern luthier.[1]

In summary, the preindustrial workflow exhibits the following strengths and weaknesses:

- Strengths
  - Lowest technological requirements
  - Highest allowance for individual creativity
  - Inherent customizability of products for end users
- Weaknesses
  - Slowest production process
  - Highest inefficiency in training, production, and use of human capital
  - Highest variability in quality.

Industrial Workflow

Technological advances of the Industrial Revolution and the widespread acceptance of the concept of (inexpensive) standardized end products led to the development of the modern industrial workflow (and society), which is characterized by homogenization of the production process, standardization of components, and exploitation of the economics of scale. In this model, products are assembled and tested via an assembly line staffed by many workers, each of whom is responsible for repeatedly performing a single, standardized task. Unlike the preindustrial workflow in which the end product is the basic unit of work, the industrial workflow embraces algorithmic analysis and subsequent pipelining of tasks into the simplest possible subtasks, with consequent elimination of a great deal of variability from the system. However, the one-size-fits-all end product allows for no creativity on the part of the assembly line workers and no ability for the customer to request product customization based on his or her preferences. Also, a shortage of one or more component can have catastrophic consequences, leading to total stoppage of the entire production line. Finally, a seemingly small change in the end product may require a large change in the production process.[2]

It is worth noting that, although the end product made using the industrial workflow can be just as complex and well-crafted as the product of a mastercrafter in the preindustrial workflow, the nature of the industrial workflow is such that the knowledge and skill to build the product is encoded in the assembly line itself as opposed to in the human beings who perform the work, leading to a sharp decrease in training requirements for workers. Near-total automation of many of the industrial processes in the late twentieth century (including that of the modern clinical chemistry laboratory) further accentuated these characteristics, frequently shifting workers from labor to essentially supervisory roles.[3] Thus, implementation of the industrial workflow can result in lower production costs, higher consistency, handling of greater volume, and, arguably, higher overall quality.

In summary, the industrial workflow exhibits the following strengths and weaknesses:

- Strengths
  - Fastest production process
  - Lowest production costs
  - High consistency
  - Capability to handle large production volumes
  - Lowest training costs for personnel

- Weaknesses
  - Low customizability
  - High barriers to process improvement
  - Talents and efforts of individuals deemphasized
  - High technological requirements.

Postindustrial Workflow

The postindustrial workflow is a natural outgrowth of the democratization of knowledge and resources made possible by the Internet and the availability of inexpensive computing hardware and software. Based largely on the work of small decentralized teams filled with highly skilled and motivated individuals, this model of workflow has been largely responsible for the success of some of today's most iconic companies (eg, Google, Facebook). Heavy use of software and computing technologies is the norm in the postindustrial workflow, and workers are expected to not only be able to use these technologies but also, at times, to have some degree of programming capability. This is because, in the postindustrial workflow, every worker is expected to be a "knowledge worker" who can provide the technical expertise for his or her own projects. As such, the postindustrial workflow has a natural fit in the technology industry, although notable nontechnology companies have also found success by following this method.[4]

   The postindustrial workflow is characterized by clusters of small, agile projects built atop a single common platform or framework, with the express goal of easy collaboration and interfacing between individual components. Teams in this setting are often encouraged to explore their own interests rather than performing only mandated roles, with a resulting increase in productivity and creativity (eg, Google's "20% Time" that allows engineers to work on projects outside their job description). At its best, the postindustrial workflow has the potential to be a truly bottom-up meritocracy in which collective decisions on an idea are made based on the strength of the idea, not on who proposed it. Because a single common platform underlies all of the disparate projects, it becomes trivially simple for even single individuals to "stand on the shoulders of giants" and synthesize new and startling uses for existing blocks of technology.

   The weaknesses of this mode of workflow relate mainly to its inability to scale past a certain point. The higher the number of people engaged in the postindustrial workflow, the more cohesion it loses, often leading to the eventual imposition of the very kinds of hierarchies that the people participating in the workflow were trying to avoid in the first place. For instance, as Google has grown in power and size, it has been unable to sustain the pure meritocracy of ideas that was its driving force at its inception. Instead, it now has adopted a corporate hierarchy that is arguably no different from that of any other corporation.[5]

   In summary, the postindustrial workflow exhibits the following strengths and weaknesses:

- Strengths
  - Fast, inexpensive production process
  - Opportunity for high individual creativity
  - Nearly infinite customizability
  - Emphasis on sharing and reuse of components leads to rapid prototyping and deployment
  - High reliability of end product, due to large progressive "standing on the shoulders of giants" effect

- Weaknesses
  - Highest technological requirements
  - Requires high technical skill from its workers
  - Lack of cohesion when scaled too high
  - Can be hostile to outsiders
  - Quality may be variable, especially when the goals of the workers and the end users do not align.

WORKFLOW AND QUALITY MANAGEMENT

No matter what mix of workflows an enterprise uses (there is arguably a place for all three workflow models in the same institution, merely in different areas), problems regarding process inefficiency and variability in end product quality are givens. Indeed, up until the 1980s, most American companies thought of quality improvement as an activity associated with driving up cost, rather than a cost-cutting measure. In hindsight, it is obvious to most observers how shortsighted a view this was. The rise of the Japanese automotive industry is now widely recognized as the triumph of those who practiced relentless quality improvement over those who scoffed at the concept. It is a story worth briefly recounting because the lessons it contains are not well understood, let alone implemented, even today.[6]

Case Study: Toyota and the Toyota Production System

The United States briefly ruled over Japan after the end of World War II. During this time, an American statistician, W. Edwards Deming, went to Japan to play a part in the 1951 Japanese census. Deming was an expert in quality control techniques and, due to his willingness to immerse himself in Japanese society, he received an invitation to work with the Japanese Union of Scientists and Engineers. Consequently, from June to August 1950, Deming trained hundreds of engineers, managers, scholars, and even top management in concepts of quality and quality control. His message to his audience would later be summarized as the "14 Points for Management"[7]:

1. Create constancy of purpose toward improvement of product and service, with the aim of becoming competitive, to stay in business, and provide jobs.
2. Adopt the new philosophy. This is the new economic age. Management must awaken to the challenge, must learn their responsibilities, and take on leadership for change.
3. Cease dependence on inspection to achieve quality. Eliminate the need for massive inspection by building quality into the product in the first place.
4. End the practice of awarding business based on a price tag. Instead, minimize total cost. Move toward a single supplier for any one item, built on a long-term relationship of trust and loyalty.
5. Improve constantly and forever the system of production and service, to improve quality and productivity, and thus constantly decrease costs.
6. Institute training on the job.
7. Institute leadership. The aim of supervision should be to help people, machines, and gadgets do a better job. Supervision of management is in need of an overhaul, as well as supervision of production workers.
8. Drive out fear, so that everyone may work effectively for the company.
9. Break down barriers between departments. People in research, design, sales, and production must work as a team, to foresee problems of production and usage that may be encountered with the product or service.

10. Eliminate slogans, exhortations, and targets for the work force that ask for zero defects and new levels of productivity. Such exhortations only create adversarial relationships because the bulk of the causes of low quality and low productivity belong to the system and thus lie beyond the power of the work force.
11. Eliminate work standards (quotas) on the factory floor. Also, eliminate management by objective (ie, with numbers and numerical goals). Substitute both with leadership.
12. Remove barriers that rob the hourly worker of his or her right to pride of workmanship. The responsibility of supervisors must be changed from generating sheer numbers to generating quality. Also, remove barriers that rob people in management and in engineering of their right to pride of workmanship. This means, among other things, the abolishment of the annual or merit rating and management by objective.
13. Institute a vigorous program of education and self-improvement.
14. Put everybody in the company to work to accomplish the transformation. The transformation is everybody's job. Massive training is required to instill the courage to break with tradition. Every activity and every job is part of the process.

Several Japanese manufacturers, including Sony, Toyota, and Yamaha, took these lessons to heart and, as a result, experienced levels of quality and productivity that had long been considered impossible in the Western world. Toyota in particular internalized Deming's philosophies, explicitly encoding them in an entity now known as the Toyota Production System (TPS). The TPS has been described as an integrated sociotechnical system that, by design, minimizes overburden (*muri*) and inconsistency (*mura*), and eliminates waste (*muda*). This depends, in turn, on the creation of a stripped-down, agile, and, above all, flexible production process that is fine-tuned and improved on by rapid iteration, with each iteration encoding more and more knowledge into (and eliminating more and more inefficiency from) the process.[8]

Waste (*muda*) is further divided into at least eight subcategories:

1. Transportation: every time a product is moved it stands the risk of being damaged, lost, or delayed. Unnecessary transportation is waste.
2. Inventory: all inventory, whether it is raw materials, works in progress, or finished but stored goods, compose a capital outlay that has not yet produced an income. Any inventory not being actively processed is waste.
3. Motion: this is the damage that the production process inflicts on the components of the production line (equipment, workers). For instance, a production process that produces a high rate of repetitive stress injury in its workers is inherently wasteful.
4. Waiting: whenever goods are not in transport or being processed, they are being wasted.
5. Overprocessing: whenever more work is done on a piece than is required, this is waste. This includes using technologies that are more precise, complex, or expensive than required.
6. Overproduction: this is the worst kind of waste. It occurs when more products are produced than are required (usually as a result of large batch processes). It can generate every other type of waste listed here.
7. Defects: these include not only products that are not within specification but also products that the customer does not want.
8. Human capital: although organizations employ staff for specific skills, these staff members may have other, often significant, skills. To not recognize and take advantage of these skills is waste.

Though many Western observers characterize the TPS as a "bottom-up" transformative process (ie, change from the bottom resulting in total cultural change), nothing could be farther from the truth.[9] The TPS is only made possible by consistent visionary leadership from the top, with the mandating of and rigorous adherence to the following at all levels[8]:

- Long-term thinking
  - Base management decisions on a long-term philosophy, even at the expense of short-term financial goals.
- Creation of the correct production process
  - Create continuous process flow to unearth problems.
  - Use a system of just-in-time production to avoid overproduction.
  - Level out the workload and do not stress any specific part (mechanical, electric, human) of the system (*heijunka*).
  - Build a culture of stopping production to fix problems to get quality right from the start.
  - Standardized tasks are the foundation for continuous incremental improvement (*kaizen*) and employee empowerment.
  - Use visual indicators (*kanban*) so no problems are hidden.
  - Use only reliable, thoroughly tested technology that serves people and processes.
- Adding value by developing people and partners
  - Grow leaders who thoroughly understand the work, live the philosophy, and teach it to others.
  - Develop exceptional people and teams that follow the philosophy.
  - Respect partners and suppliers by challenging them and helping them improve.
- Organizational learning by continuously confronting root problems
  - Go and see for yourself to thoroughly understand the situation (*genchi genbutsu*).
  - Make decisions slowly by consensus, thoroughly considering all options; however, implement decisions rapidly (*nemawashi*).
  - Focus always on relentless reflection (*hansei*) and improvement (*kaizen*).

As a result, Toyota was able to reduce cost and lead-time (ie, the time between the placement of an order and delivery) while simultaneously and dramatically improving quality over time. Accordingly, it became the largest car manufacturer in the world by 2007 and more profitable than all the other car companies in the world combined.[10]

Compare this to the actions and reactions of the American car industry over the course of most of the last half-century. Quality improvement was seen as a cost-inflating measurement and was avoided by workers and management except when absolutely necessary. Complacency and arrogance created a culture in which creative thinking and teamwork were discouraged. In the meantime, American cars could no longer compete with Japanese cars on quality, so they were forced to compete instead on price, driving down American car quality even further. By the early 1980s, the era of American dominance in the car industry was arguably over, and American car manufacturers were grudgingly forced to begin adopting Toyota-style production quality improvement measures. As a final note, a system like the TPS only works so long as it is (1) culturally ingrained and (2) rigorously followed. This requires significant investment in the company on the part of the workers, with an unfailing pursuit of quality above all else (at which even Toyota failed recently).[11]

Finally, there exists an offshoot of the TPS known as Lean. It is not as rigidly defined as the TPS and is best understood as a generalization of the TPS principles into industries other than manufacturing. As such, it has only two key differences in practice[12]:

- Although seeking profit is perhaps the key focus of the TPS, Lean implementations tend to deemphasize this, instead seeking process improvement for other reasons specific to the industry or organization.
- In the TPS, the area of skills development is that of the work team leader, and not a trained TPS specialist. In Lean, this is often reversed: emphasis is placed on developing the specialist, whereas work team leader skill development is less emphasized.

Case Study: Motorola, General Electric, and Six Sigma

Like the TPS-Lean, Six Sigma is a Deming-inspired business management strategy that seeks to eliminate defects and reduce process variation. Six Sigma, however, differs from TPS in the following ways[13]:

- All Six Sigma projects must achieve a measurable and quantifiable financial return.
- Six Sigma requires a special infrastructure of Six Sigma experts (named after belt colors in martial arts) to lead and implement projects.
- Decisions are made only based on verifiable data, instead of than on assumptions and guesswork.

The end goal of a Six Sigma project is to produce most end products within specification. This is accepted to mean less than one defect per million opportunities (DPMO) in the short-term, and approximately 3.4 DPMO in the long term. The name "Six Sigma" itself comes from recognition that if one has at least six standard deviations between the process mean and the nearest specification limit, zero items will fail to meet specifications. Unfortunately, it has also been recognized that processes tend to regress in quality control over time, settling on a mean of 4.5 deviations between the process mean and the nearest specification limit on the long term (which explains why 3.4 DPMO in the long term is still considered a Six Sigma success).[13]

Developed by Motorola in 1986 and championed at General Electric by Jack Welch in the 1990s, Six Sigma initially raised a great deal of interest, perhaps largely because of the tremendous savings that these two companies initially reported as a direct result of implementing Six Sigma. By the late 1990s, Six Sigma had become so popular that about two-thirds of the Fortune 500 organizations had adopted Six Sigma as standard operating procedure. It is unfortunately telling that (1) 91% of these companies that adopted Six Sigma have trailed the Standard & Poor (S&P) 500 ever since,[14] (2) well-documented, peer-reviewed evidence for Six Sigma success is relatively rare, and (3) Motorola itself failed to adapt to the disruptive change that Apple brought to the telecommunication industry in the form of the iPhone. As a result, it has performed so poorly in recent years that it had to be split into two independent companies—one of which was recently bought by Google largely for the value of its intellectual property and the other of which only continues in a much diminished capacity.[15]

Though there may be a case for the short-term benefits of Six Sigma as narrowly applied to an existing production process, the long-term benefits of Six Sigma from an organizational standpoint are unclear at best and nonexistent at worst. It is not known why this is the case. What can be observed, however, is that even though

Six Sigma claims to be an improvement on Deming's by-now battle-tested philosophies, it actually disregards several of Deming's most important rules:

- Six Sigma is by nature a zero-defect-type policy, entirely disregarding point 10 of Deming's "14 Points for Management."
- Six Sigma focuses on measurable outcomes and short-term profits, entirely disregarding points 11 and 12 of Deming's "14 Points for Management."
- Six Sigma relies on specific actors ("Black Belts") to drive change, entirely disregarding points 13 and 14 of Deming's "14 Points for Management."
- Perhaps most importantly, Six Sigma is driven by data, not knowledge. This has the effect of stifling creativity and necessitating a rigid production process, which is the exact opposite of the ideal production process that Deming championed. A Six Sigma production process may thus be optimized for the present, but it runs the danger of being woefully unprepared for the future.

PATHOLOGY PRODUCTION PROCESSES

The pathology workflow can generally be defined as the process by which a certain raw material (eg, human cerebrospinal fluid or tissue) is converted into a certain end product, such as a laboratory test result or pathology report (data) to provide information for actionable clinical knowledge. Since the specifics of any given production process are largely dependent on the nature of (1) the raw material and (2) the desired end product, it should come as no surprise that different pathology subspecialties have somewhat different associated workflows. However, all pathology workflows have the following characteristics in common:

- They can broadly be broken down into three phases:
  - Preanalytic
  - Analytic
  - Postanalytic
- They consist of a series of intermediate steps of variable complexity:
  - Some steps can be automated
    - Example: uncapping of a standard blood tube (in chemistry)
    - Example: printout of a labeled cassette (in surgical pathology)
  - Some steps follow a rigid algorithm, but require human intervention
    - Example: preparing a nonstandard microbiology specimen (in microbial pathology)
    - Example: case assembly (in surgical pathology)
  - Some steps require much attention and work by a skilled artisan
    - Example: examination of morphologic patterns (in hematology, immunopathology cytology)
    - Example: sign-out (in surgical pathology, cytopathology, hematopathology)
- They have certain unavoidable waiting periods built-in
  - Example: formalin fixation time (in surgical pathology)
  - Example: polymerase chain reaction amplification time (in molecular pathology)
- Supported by highly-complex production management software packages known collectively as laboratory information systems (LIS).[16]

At present, information systems that include the clinical pathology (CP) laboratory information system (CPLIS), the anatomic pathology (AP) laboratory information system (APLIS), and the electronic medical record (EMR) systems, are predominantly monolithic units sold by individual vendors who have little interest in providing the end user with flexibility or interoperability (even among products sold and supported by the same vendor). As such, workflow improvement projects in pathology (and indeed in medicine in general) are almost always as much about working around the rigid limitations of these information systems as they are about actual improvement in workflow. This is one of the greatest ironies (and tragedies) of this development: pathologists have, in a very real sense, become slaves to the very systems that supposedly make their and their patients' lives easier.

AP

AP has, largely due to the nature and lower volume of its specimens and the hands-on operations that must be performed on some of those specimens, traditionally lagged behind CP in its automation of workflow. With the relatively recent advent of technologies such as bar coding and radiofrequency identification (RFID) tagging, new possibilities for improvement in AP workflow have opened up. Indeed, certain pathology departments (most notably the Henry Ford Hospital System, Detroit, Michigan, USA)[17] have developed and adopted quality management programs that bear a striking resemblance to the TPS (as previously discussed). There is much to learn from the successes and, just as important, the failures of these quality management programs. The following section focuses on the generalized AP workflow (its preanalytic, analytic, and postanalytic phases) while noting areas for (and barriers to) possible workflow improvement.

AP: preanalytic phase

Although with a contemporary CPLIS or APLIS most orders are handled by a computerized provider order entry (CPOE) system, for the APLIS the order entry is still largely manual and dependent on paper, often with handwritten requisitions. When implemented in a fashion that allows free electronic interchange of clinical data between the APLIS and the upstream ordering EMR systems, CPOE can unlock a wide variety of benefits, including but not limited to[18]:

- Reduced turnaround time
- Reduced manual steps, including transcription, label writing, and accessioning
- Elimination of ambiguous and/or indecipherable orders
- Improved compliance with laboratory testing and/or clinical guidelines
- Improved test use
- Improved appropriateness of test ordering.

Although it is beyond the scope of this article to provide a full discussion of CPOE and its implementation, it is important for the pathologist to understand why CPOE is not commonly implemented in AP:

- There are no specific dictionary-driven tests (eg, serum glucose, 24-hour urine protein) in CP; specimens are generically called surgical pathology, cytopathology, or autopsy specimens.
- AP orders often require more information compared with CP orders; a blood specimen for chemistry testing can simply be specified by checking off the appropriate box for the desired testing, whereas an AP order would ideally contain information such as an organ of origin, specific demographic data, and relevant clinical information.
- A single AP order may encompass several parts from several different organs; this is not something that CP has to commonly deal with.
- AP specimen collection is inherently procedure-driven as opposed to CP specimens, which often require nothing more than a blood draw. For instance, a surgeon might initially place an order for an AP specimen but later be either

unable or unwilling to collect the specimen because of operation complexity or patient instability.
- There is a paucity of vendors with AP systems that currently support CPOE.

The first interaction an APLIS usually has with a specimen is at the time of its receipt in the AP laboratory, usually with a printed requisition. Once the case is received, a human is required to manually accession the case, during which (1) the APLIS assigns it a unique accession number and (2) related information from the requisition is entered into the APLIS. In multipart cases, each part is entered and documented separately.

There are two data fields in particular that are important at this stage: the part type and the part description. The part type is chosen from the possible specimen types that have been built into the APLIS part-type dictionary and cannot be entered as free text. Other data fields, including fee codes and histology protocols, can be auto-populated given the part type. For instance, a part type of "stomach biopsy" might trigger a histology protocol for hematoxylin-eosin stain, magnification 3, and an immunohistochemical stain protocol for *Helicobacter pylori*. In contrast, the part description is most often a free-text field. It comprises the descriptive information about the specimen that was provided in the requisition (eg, left breast mastectomy). Although this information, like any free-text field, currently has no bearing on the automated processes of a present-day APLIS, it can provide important information to the pathologist interpreting the case. For each specimen, the corresponding information about the patient (eg, demographics, billing details, home address) can either be entered into the APLIS programmatically (typically via an admit-discharge-transfer feed transmitted from the upstream hospital information system) or manually by an accessioner. The latter is inherently prone to more errors.

Workflow improvement in the preanalytic phase encounters a many barriers, largely because it inherently involves the handoff of a medicolegal entity (the specimen) from one system with a very specific set of priorities (provided by the surgery team) to another system with an often very different set of priorities (those of the AP team). Moreover, the AP team often does not own much of the preanalytic workflow process. In the operating room, information critical to proper handling of the specimen is recorded by individuals who (1) are not doctors and (2) often have no training in pathology. These individuals cannot be expected to understand what clinical information would be most relevant to the downstream pathologist. Errors that arise from this, including improper labeling, orientation and/or fixation of specimens, are often beyond the power of the AP team to catch at the time they are made, unless the team took the unprecedented step of embedding someone trained in properly accessioning and orienting specimens in every operating room from which specimens were received. Though this would have obvious benefits, the labor costs, especially in large facilities with numerous operating rooms, is prohibitively high.

Additional serious difficulties in implementing CPOE are largely related to the inflexibility of the upstream (the surgical component of the EMR) and the downstream (the APLIS) systems. Ideally, the CPOE system would autogenerate specimen labels with bar coding and/or RFID tagging native to the APLIS in a just-in-time basis for specimen collection (which is standard of care with CPLIS), but this would require (1) giving the EMR the power to make the APLIS automatically generate an accession number for the case, (2) algorithmically matching the part description (which is what the surgeon tells the nurse to call the specimen at the time of collection) with the appropriate part type (which is a much more rigidly defined element in the APLIS) with accuracy, (3) making sure the relevant (and only the relevant) clinical data was included on or with the requisition, and (4) making sure the accession class is correct (a problem found in large systems with subspecialty sign-out, in which a specimen collected at one hospital may need to be accessioned to and examined at the AP laboratory of an entirely different hospital).

AP: analytic phase

Gross examination Once the preanalytic phase is over, the case status is updated to accessioned. At this point, the specimen enters the hands of the prosector who will perform the first part of the analytic phase. The first part of this phase, gross examination (often referred to as grossing), involves the description of the gross appearance of the specimen, dissection of the specimen, selection of individual tissue sections, and designation of these sections for microscopic examination. Gross descriptions are mainly done in free text, usually by way of dictated description. Text templates for commonly processed specimen types exist (eg, small biopsies) and there have been some successes with speech-to-text recognition software at this stage.[16]

The final product of the first part of this phase is the so-called gross report, which consists of a description of the specimen, how it was dissected, what was seen macroscopically on dissection, and a key (ie, alphanumeric list) designating what tissue went into each cassette. This key becomes important to the APLIS at this point. However, in the absence of truly effective natural language parsing algorithms that could render a gross report into machine-understandable form, it is currently impossible to programmatically extract clinically useful information from the report. Cassette engravers may be interfaced with the APLIS to keep track of how many tissue cassettes were made per case, but do not provide meaningful information on the kind of tissue that went into the cassette. As such, tissue cassette designations must usually be entered into the APLIS by hand. Gross specimen digital images may be commonly acquired during grossing, and some APLISs have integrated modules to accommodate and manage those images.[16]

There are several possibilities for workflow improvement at this stage. Although it is true that each specimen is unique, it is also true that the specific way a specimen is grossed is entirely dependent on the skills and inclinations of the prosector. This is the root of most of the workflow issues that arise herein—the grossing step is mainly preindustrial and artisanal in nature, and is largely resistant to change. The question of how many sections are enough for a given specimen has been the subject of lively debate since the dawn of pathology as a medical discipline, but most institutions have at least informal rules on how large specimens are to be grossed. A single universal consensus standard in this respect is desirable for the purposes of workflow, but may not be attainable for multiple (largely political) reasons.

Bar coding and other unique identification technologies enter into the picture at the time of case accessioning, but also have applications in the grossing step. A certain number of bar coded and prenumbered cassettes can be automatically generated given the part type (for instance, a routine colonic biopsy would usually require only one cassette). Barcodes on the specimen requisition or the specimen container can be used as an identifier of the specimen for the APLIS or to the gross photograph management system (if that system is not part of the APLIS), reducing errors in the photography phase. These identification technologies can also theoretically be used to enable truly granular tracking of the case through the grossing phase, but this is not usually done for reasons ranging from the technical (an inflexible APLIS that does not provide facilities for such asset tracking) to the pragmatic (the labor costs of such granular tracking may not justify the possible benefit).[19]

Synoptic grossing is the idea that a gross report can be divided into discrete data elements in the fashion of synoptic reporting of cancer specimens (which is now becoming de rigueur in AP). The difficulty in doing this lies in part with the inflexibility of the APLIS, but also in part because different pieces of data are important for different specimens. The measurements that are important for a uterus removed for leiomyomata are very different from those important for a uterus removed for confirmed papillary serous carcinoma and, indeed, a uterus removed for leiomyomata may incidentally be found to be harboring a carcinoma. Furthermore, the measurements taken during gross examination are usually less accurate than measurements taken during microscopic examination and, as such, are accorded a place of lesser importance.

However, there are several places (most notably in autopsy pathology) where gross measurement is still of great importance. In autopsy pathology, measurements of size and weight can considerably affect the final diagnosis, especially if the decedent is perinatal. In addition, autopsy pathology involves the generation of extremely long gross descriptions that can largely be templated and standardized on an institution-by-institution basis. As such, autopsy pathology provides the ideal use case for synoptic grossing and, to the best of the authors' knowledge, at least one major hospital system in the USA has a pilot project for the use of synoptic grossing in perinatal autopsies in development.

Finally, there is the more mundane, yet critically important, matter of supply-chain logistics for the gross examination room. For a gross examination room to operate in an optimal fashion, the necessary equipment (eg, scalpels, forceps, formalin) must be present in sufficient quantity and condition. Too much or idiosyncratically sorted equipment leads to clutter and confusion, decreasing the overall efficiency of the gross examination room. On the other hand, the absence of proper equipment disrupts the workflow of gross examination altogether, leading to suboptimal grossing at best and a total stoppage of workflow at worst. It is entirely possible to implement just-in-time supply chain logistics for this area of the AP laboratory; however, this is an issue that traditionally has been ignored. Moreover, a system needs to be in place to be able to readily retrieve already grossed, stored specimens to submit additional tissue sections, use them for teaching purposes, and so forth, before they are discarded.

Tissue processing The histology (or the cytology) laboratory, because of its assembly line nature, is the target of many process improvement projects. Slide labels are now often autogenerated based on the tissue cassette data previously entered by the prosector. Specimen tracking and bar coding are being increasingly used in this phase, with the LIS providing the ability to update specimen status and location based on the scanning of a bar code, or, less frequently, an RFID-enabled tag. Some APLISs have gone as far as to autogenerate bar coded and labeled slides at individual histotechnologist stations at the time of individual case microtomy, leading to a reduction in case misidentification and an improvement in histotechnologist efficiency. Once the slides have been created and are ready for distribution, the slides are often paired with an autogenerated paper working draft (so-called case assembly), which is templated within the APLIS and includes requisition data, the patient's demographics and relevant clinical history, the gross description of the specimen, any intraoperative consultation diagnosis, and the patient's past AP reports. Efforts in several laboratories are underway to become paperless and, thereby, avoid this error-prone manual, matching case assembly step.

Many laboratories have reported on the rigorous usage of bar coding in this phase, all reporting large decreases in mislabeled blocks and slides, and some reporting decreases in turnaround time. This comes as no surprise; the histology laboratory has traditionally been the part of the AP workflow that bears the largest similarities to a standard manufacturing production process. Implementations of TPS-like cultures of continual improvement focus on this area of AP heavily, with the goal of eliminating many sources of waste (*muda*) from the production line. For example, in 2008 the University of Pittsburgh Medical Center Shadyside Hospital (Pittsburgh, PA, USA) histology laboratory found that specimens were undergoing excessive transportation during the production process. By rearranging laboratory equipment and reconfiguring the phases of production, the laboratory team (1) drastically reduced the transportation individual specimens underwent and (2) simplified the assembly line in the process, with a resultant 21% decrease in specimen processing time.[20]

Case assembly provides the first logical point in the system for scanning of slides as whole slide images (WSI). It is possible that, eventually, all AP laboratories will operate in a slideless fashion, with primary diagnoses being rendered using WSI instead of the source glass slides. Currently, (1) no WSI system is FDA-approved for primary diagnosis, (2) WSI is not currently widely used for cytopathology and hematopathology, and (3) scanning times are still far too long for a single WSI scanner to be able to serve the needs of even a moderate-volume service, A batch of 120 slides, a mere six trays, take 2 hours minimum to scan, even with the fastest scanner on the market. As such, it is currently unlikely for WSI to be considered as a workflow improvement at the time of case assembly. See the discussion by Seung Park and colleagues elsewhere in this issue of the pros and cons of WSI.

Finally, as in the case for the gross examination room, there is the issue of supply chain logistics for the histology and cytology laboratory. Traditionally, tissue processing laboratories choose to err on the side of overstocking raw materials, with the resultant problems of a more disorganized workspace and occasional expiration of reagents. Just as in the gross examination room, just-in-time supply chain logistics with heavy usage of visual indicators (*kanban*) would theoretically have the effect of reducing the waste of space (due to excess raw material on hand) and time (due to the resultant clutter of the workspace), but such projects are rarely, if ever, reported in the literature.

Microscopic examination and sign-out Once a case has reached the pathologist, the analytic phase nears its end. If at this point the pathologist needs to order recuts (additional hematoxylin-eosin stained slides), special stains, immunohistochemical stains, or other studies before making his or her diagnosis, this can be done either through paper requisitions or through a CPOE interface. Final pathologic diagnosis, such as gross examination, in most institutions is largely a free-text affair, usually involving transcription of a pathologist's dictation. Just as in gross examination, other options include selection of predefined templates or Quicktext for frequent diagnoses (eg, hyperplastic polyp) by using either dropdown lists or coded text entry, and/or speech-to-text conversion by voice recognition software. Once the final diagnosis has been entered, the case is marked as final in the APLIS and then placed on the pathologist's queue (work list) for final edits and electronic sign-out. Billing and diagnostic codes are often entered automatically at this point, based on part type, stain orders, and, sometimes, rudimentary natural language processing of the final report.

This phase is an area of intense interest for workflow improvement, largely because anatomic pathologists are traditionally the highest-paid individuals in the clinical laboratory, thus their time is an extremely precious commodity. Any improvement that can be made to help pathologists save time and effort in this phase, therefore, should be seriously considered. Moreover, because most medicolegal errors arise from errors in the analytic phase, this is a crucial component of the test process for quality improvement intervention. Much current work, in academia and in industry, has focused on the use of WSI as the basis for advances in pathologist workflow. Some of the advantages of a WSI-based workflow, including that, in a slideless laboratory, it is impossible for slides to be lost or misplaced, are immediately obvious. However, others, including the possibility of creating an entirely new user interface model that would bring disruptive change to the workflow in the way that Apple's iPhone disrupted the Smartphone industry, have been harder to grasp, let alone implement.[21] See the article by Seung Park and colleagues elsewhere in this issue for a fuller discussion of WSI and its possibilities in pathology workflow.

Bar coded tracking of slides usually completely breaks down in this phase due to the common perception that it is not good use of a pathologist's time to be bar code scanning all slides. Therefore, it becomes impossible to know exactly where a slide is once it has left the histology laboratory. To make matters worse, the most interesting slides of a case are the ones that are most likely to be shown to other pathologists for the purposes of teaching, consultation, and quality assurance. As a result, it is common for the slides most critical for the diagnosis of a case to go missing and, for many people, including other pathologists, to be enlisted in the hunt for those slides. This represents a quantifiable waste of time and the irretrievable loss of critical patient data. On the other hand, there are serious objections to the use of pathologists as data capture points for asset tracking. The potential benefits may not justify the costs, monetary and human, and it is uncertain that compliance with such a mandate would be very high.

Because so much AP data are stored as narrative free text, it is not as easy to analyze the data in an APLIS as it is in a CPLIS. Not surprisingly, there is an increased push toward the deconvolution of text-based pathology reports into more structured synoptic reports that contain discrete data elements. Use of synoptic checklists makes reporting efficient, uniform, and complete. Synoptic checklists can be customized by individual laboratories to incorporate,–and potentially track, data elements important to their practices. Several LISs offer synoptic reporting modules, and there are third-party synoptic reporting programs that are made to interface with LISs that do not have those capabilities built in. The discrete data elements contained in synoptic reports can theoretically be analyzed at will, resulting in facilitated quality assurance and research initiatives.[22]

Finally, it should not be forgotten that, though it is likely that standardized synoptic reporting is the future of surgical pathology sign-out, in its current state the pathologist's workflow is inherently preindustrial and artisanal in nature. This is reflected in the way that pathologists, and all physicians, are trained: as apprentices to master physicians who impart their skills and knowledge in the manner of the mastercrafters of old. There are elements of this workflow that have never been, and perhaps will never be, studied because they are simply culturally accepted as the norm. For example, the reasons why pathologists receive their cases in batches, instead of one-by-one in a just-in-time basis, are as much cultural as they are technical. It will likely take the presence of a disruptive external force for this profession as a whole to seriously reevaluate the merits of our current artisanal sign-out system.

AP: postanalytic phase

The postanalytic phase is traditionally when quality assurance and research initiatives take place. This phase enjoys the lack of certain time pressures, in that the cases are already signed out (the actionable clinical data has been delivered to the clinicians). It is possible to implement the automated flagging of cases for randomized quality assurance review within the APLIS, removing the need for a human to do such flagging. It is likewise possible, because of the small percentage of cases that undergo such review, to do such flagging during the preanalytic phase and selectively scan those cases as WSIs. This allows for (1) minimal disturbance in case turnaround time given the small number of slides to be scanned, even with the current speed of WSI scanners and (2) immediate access to digital slides for review instead of the current situation, in which someone has to find the glass slides and then hand them off to the reviewing pathologist.

Amendments and addenda are an unfortunate fact of life in the AP realm and, as such, the APLIS must be flexible enough to handle these postanalytic reporting events. It is desirable for the system to capture the reason for the issuance of any given amendment or addendum as a discrete data element for both documentation and business analytics purposes. This is usually done by defining a list of accepted reasons for an amendment or an addendum within the APLIS and by requiring pathologists to choose a valid reason from that list when creating an amendment or an addendum.

Educational efforts in the postanalytic phase largely revolve around compilation of interesting slides into teaching sets, and the ordering of recuts for individual residents. Both endeavors benefit greatly from the use of WSI, especially in the case of educational recuts; these could be considered a waste of time and resources in the presence of acceptable digital alternatives. Increasingly, proficiency tests such as those offered by the College of American Pathologists are including digital slides. Currently, these digital slides are offered in addition to the glass slides, but it is clear that, at some point in the future, digital slides will be the only modality offered.

AP: cytopathology

Cytopathology presents unique challenges and unique opportunities in this domain. The workflow of cytopathology is unlike that of surgical pathology because the prepared slides are first sent to cytotechnologists who screen the slides for the pathologists. Therefore, some APLISs allow separate fields for screener impressions and final diagnosis. Cytopathology requires an assessment of whether the obtained specimen is adequate (satisfactory or unsatisfactory), a primary interpretation (negative, atypical, suspicious, positive), as well as a final diagnosis. This must all be designed into the APLIS. Gynecologic and thyroid cytopathology have codified diagnostic terminologies (the Bethesda System), which have paved the way for a future in which diagnosis in cytopathology will become increasingly standardized. Although this creates added complexity in APLIS design, it also allows for increasing amounts of cytopathology data to be held as discrete data elements instead of as free text. This fact allows for easier statistical analysis of current cytopathology diagnostic data and has wide-ranging implications for cytopathology data mining. Furthermore, in certain circumstances a particular diagnosis (eg, atypical cells of undetermined significance on a peroxidase-antiperoxidase [PAP] test) might lead to reflex testing (eg, high-risk human papillomavirus). This, too, could be built into the APLIS.

There are screening and performance indicators mandated by law (ie, CLIA 1988) that must be considered. Provisions for setting up the maximum workload for individual cytotechnologists are one such consideration. United States federal law requires that cytotechnologists manually document the number of slides screened in each 24-hour period and the number of hours spent screening each day. It is illegal to screen more than 100 slides per 8-hour period or 12.5 slides per hour. The LIS could keep track of these things and lock out individual cytotechnologists once their case limits have been reached. Another consideration is the practice of rescreening. At a minimum, in the United States a 10% random rescreen of negative PAP stains and a rescreening of a specific percentage of negative "high risk" cases are mandatory. This, however, does not take into account that different users might require different rescreening measures. For instance, a cytotechnologist fresh out of training may require a higher rescreening ratio than a cytotechnologist with 30 years' experience. The LIS can be instrumental in setting up these individual thresholds. Furthermore, the LIS can be used to ensure that each practitioner, and the practice as a whole, is doing appropriate rescreening.

The LIS could also be used to automatically flag cases which would traditionally be described as high risk because of previous history or current history of abnormal signs, symptoms, and/or pathologic findings. This can involve natural language parsing of free-text fields such as "clinical history" and "case description" with the goal of searching for suspicious text strings such as "history of LSIL." It can also involve the presence of previous cases such as a PAP smear that was diagnosed with LSIL the previous year. By using an algorithm (tuned to the specific laboratory) on all gynecologic cytology cases, the LIS can automatically alert the pathologist to cases that fall under its high risk criteria, thus improving both patient care and turnaround time.[23]

AP: role of the APLIS

Even a cursory examination of the relationship between the anatomic pathologist and the APLIS that he or she uses reveals two uncomfortable truths:

- The pathologist is largely dependent on the APLIS to provide the level of service to which our clinicians and patients are accustomed.
- The pathologist often struggles with the user interface of the APLIS.

This dichotomy occurs because modern APLISs are, by and large, proprietary systems built by companies that have historically taken a narrow view on what the functionality of an APLIS should be. The companies are not wholly to blame; after all, the APLIS has been asked, variously, to be:

- An order entry system
- An asset tracking system
- A billing system
- A quality assurance system
- An image management system
- A business analytics system.

Every single item on that bullet list represents a disparate entity with unique performance and user interface requirements. It is perhaps unfair to ask modern APLISs, whose design characteristics were largely defined in the 1980s, to be able to take on all those roles at once. Indeed, the act of modifying an APLIS to support a role that it was not initially designed to support is generally a tedious and arduous endeavor requiring hundreds of person-hours to successfully complete.

However, this does not change that our workflow is often as defined by what the APLIS cannot do as it is by what it can do. From the human-computer interaction literature, it is known that a better user interface can provide massive savings in end-user time and, in the AP community, it is known that the user interfaces of modern APLISs can be described as mediocre at best. It is strange that more work has not, up until very recently, been done in this area.

CP

CP, on the other hand, represents the pinnacle of automation in modern medicine. Though it started historically at the same point as AP, when all tests had to be performed by hand, it has reached a point at which sophisticated analytic machines that mostly operate without human intervention are responsible for most tests performed in the modern clinical laboratory. The reasons for are that most clinical laboratory tests are qualitative or quantitative, but not narrative, in nature, meaning that these tests can be analyzed, interpreted, and stored as discrete data elements.[24]

Automation has been applied to the preanalytic, analytic, and postanalytic stages of laboratory testing. Today, commercial total laboratory automation (TLA) systems are used in many hospital-based laboratories; these (1) couple several instruments to an integrated specimen management and transportation system, and (2) involve process control software that is seamlessly linked to, or even a part of, the CPLIS. Though standards in TLA have emerged over the years, there are still great technical and engineering hurdles to overcome in developing and implementing such a system, mostly related to the integration of disparate systems (including commercial laboratory instruments and user-defined work cells). Other factors that need to be taken into consideration include selecting the best-fit automation system for a laboratory, the capabilities of the existing LIS, operation cost, test-volume growth potential, process improvement, patient safety, and facilities infrastructure.[25]

CP: preanalytic phase

This phase focuses on specimen transportation and sample processing. Relying on courier services to deliver specimens to the laboratory relies on a batch process and is often plagued by staffing and/or scheduling issues. Some laboratories have explored using mobile robotic vehicles for transportation of patient specimens, while others use computer-controlled pneumatic tube networks. These approaches have all been shown to reduce the turnaround time of results. However, pneumatic tubes can subject specimens to rapid acceleration and deceleration, which may have unintended effects on specimens (eg, hemolysis in extreme cases).[26]

With the advent of point-of-care testing (POCT), fewer specimens are now sent to the central laboratory. POCT devices are often preferred by clinical staff for their ease of use and their very fast turnaround time as opposed to traditional central laboratory testing. Some institutions have even created a remotely controlled automated clinical laboratory that provides testing near the patient's bedside, while maintaining the distinct advantage of central laboratory control.[27]

Unlike in the APLIS, in the CPLIS specimens can be accessioned before they ever come to the laboratory. If the upstream EMR's CPOE subsystem has order communication to the LIS, then the order is electronically transferred to the LIS, which automatically generates an accession number for the case and arranges for a specimen tube label with bar coding innate to the LIS to be generated at or near the patient care area (either immediately in the case of stat laboratory tests or as part of a batch in the case of routine laboratory test). This, in conjunction with other positive patient identification techniques, has the effect of reducing error in specimen collection.

After arriving in the laboratory, several tasks need to be accomplished with specimens, including identification, labeling, sorting, centrifuging, decapping, aliquoting, recapping, and storage. If performed manually, these steps are fraught with potential safety hazards and risk for errors, and may cause potential delays in test processing. Fortunately, at least in the modern clinical chemistry laboratory, almost all of the above steps have been automated. Laboratories have the choice of using several standalone automated units (each of which might perform some of the above tasks) or a single modular hands-free system that automates the entire process. However, similar automation in other areas of CP are less well developed and in need of sustained developmental efforts.

CP: analytic phase

The analytic phase requires tubes to be directly placed onto instruments (AutoAnalyzers). Contemporary instruments have consolidated most high-volume tests into a single platform, offering a large menu of varied assays. Such analyzers produce high specimen throughput rates yet provide great flexibility for random access testing. These analyzers feature onboard computers linked to sophisticated arrays of sensors and robotic platforms that cannot only optimally perform each test every single time, but can also track reagents in real time, offer troubleshooting, and provide training protocols.

Several automated instruments use digital imaging techniques no less sophisticated than those being used in AP. Such instruments may contain a camera station capable of recognizing different tubes, sample material, and performing sample volume calculations. Certain hematology analyzers (eg, CellaVision DM1200, BloodHound Integrated Hematology System) even integrate full-featured WSI capabilities, leveraging those capabilities in automated microscopic analysis, quick review, and even telepathology.

Instruments harbor their own on-board computer that is linked to the LIS or some other master controller computer system. These systems can have either unidirectional or bidirectional interfaces with the LIS. In a unidirectional interface, the laboratory technologist manually enters test orders on the device. After the analysis, the results are transmitted electronically to the LIS. With a bidirectional interface, on the other hand, the LIS transmits the test order to the device and also receives the final results. Electronic test orders can be transmitted to instruments either (1) directly on receipt or entry of the order in the LIS (broadcast type) or (2) when a tube gets placed on the analyzers (query type). For the latter interface, reading of the bar code on the specimen tube by the analyzer triggers a query to the LIS for any orders related to that accession number.

The act of linking instrument computers to the LIS had a profound impact on automation in the clinical laboratory. For example, the LIS can easily perform calculations (eg, delta checks) and execute algorithms, reflex testing, or rules. Many of these rely on rule-based logic—an algorithmic set of steps that execute based on programmatic control statements (eg, if or then) that perform comparisons on a specific base state. This improves productivity and consistency, reduces the need for staff, lowers errors, and speeds up workflow. Perhaps the most popular example of rule-based logic at work is autoverification. Autoverification refers to the automatic review and verification of results received from a laboratory instrument without the intervention of a technologist. In autoverification, a test result transmitted over an instrument interface is either passed or failed by the LIS, based on parameters that the laboratory defines for its system. If it passes, the result is autoverified and no human intervention is required. If it fails, the test is flagged for manual review by a technologist. The Clinical and Laboratory Standards Institute has published guidelines for autoverification (AUTO 10A). Autoverification rules and process must be tested at least annually to be in compliance with regulatory requirements.[28]

CP: postanalytic phase

The postanalytic phase involves the delivery of diagnostic information to health care providers and the storage of specimens. The topic of electronic transmission of test results from the LIS to the upstream EMR is beyond the scope of this article; however, it should be recognized as an important form of automation without which the clinical laboratory simply could not support high-volume testing. Specimen storage and tracking systems can also produce large gains in productivity and use sophisticated robotics to do so efficiently; some studies suggest that these systems can reduce the time to find a sample by as much as 60%. Some storage systems even have facilities for automatic sample disposal at predetermined times.[29]

FUTURE TRENDS AND SUMMARY

This is a time of great excitement and opportunity for the discipline of pathology. Advances in genomic, molecular diagnostic, imaging, and data analytic techniques have allowed—perhaps for the first time—a glimpse into a future in which hidden patterns embedded in our visual (eg, WSI) and numerical (eg, laboratory tests) data will be brought to light that can be exploited for the benefit of the patient.[30–32] For pathologists to face the challenges, and capitalize on the opportunities, that the so-called digital decade of personalized medicine will bring, it is imperative to find ways to make the data systems transparently interoperable. Unfortunately, the pathology community is significantly hindered because most institutions have already made significant investments in LIS and EMR systems that are proprietary and for the most part closed, with even small interoperability projects requiring large investments in engineering and vendor support to complete. These systems may adequately serve the needs of our hospital systems as they have traditionally existed, but they are too rigid and not interoperable for the realities of a world in which patients, computer-aided diagnostic modalities, and analytic algorithms will all demand access to flexible clinical data on a real-time basis.

The EMR and, as part of it, the APLIS and CPLIS, of the future will be gauged not by how easy it is to put clinical information into the system but by how easy it is to extract meaningful data out of the system (and perform analyses on that data). Indeed, several of the criteria and requirements in the meaningful use of EMRs relate directly or indirectly to laboratory testing and laboratory information management.[33] These future medical information systems will enable a truly postindustrial workflow, in which (1) patients may have real-time access to the very same EMR systems their doctors use and (2) real-time analytics platforms can be easily built by small teams of individuals atop the foundations laid by truly interoperable EMRs with open application programming interfaces for the retrieval and manipulation of patient data. It is preferable that pathologists take at least small steps toward such EMRs and LISs now; otherwise, outside forces (eg, pressure from society, commercial entities, legislation) will inevitably force us to do so in a manner and timeframe not of our choosing. Indeed, aspects of such approaches are already being pursued by direct-to-consumer genomics companies.[34] Because it is true that one LIS cannot be simply dropped in as a replacement for another, time and resources may need to be spent creating middleware solutions that will eventually serve as (1) the basis of the EMR and LIS of tomorrow and (2) a compatibility layer in between present and future EMRs and LISs. This strategy has the advantage of not disrupting clinical care as it stands today, while allowing data to be liberated from their prisons in the current rigid and not interoperable EMRs and LISs.

As a corollary to this, it is imperative that pathologists participate in public and corporate discourse on the present and future of the EMR and LIS today. Just as an army is guaranteed to lose 100% of the battles for which it does not show up, pathologists are guaranteed to be given less and less mindshare over time if we do not make the fate of our overarching EMR systems one of our top priorities. It is imperative that we do this because, as this article demonstrates, our information systems in large part determine our workflows. We have allowed our workflows to become suboptimal because we have ceded control of these computerized systems to companies that historically have not understood (1) what the workflow of pathology (and medicine in general) is and, more importantly, (2) what the workflow of pathology (and medicine in general) could optimally be.

Pathologists must be the champions of positive change in workflow and implementation of electronic health records in our institutions and in medicine at large. It is inevitable that the data within our laboratory information systems will be opened up for real-time data analysis and clinical decision support. It is also inevitable that our workflow will have to change, sometimes radically, in response to the demands of the digital decade of personalized medicine before us. We can be visionary leaders and drivers of workflow change. In doing so, we have the opportunity to take the destiny of medicine into our hands. Or we can be content to be followers or even to ignore the disruptive changes that loom before us; this being the path of diminishment and relegation to eventual irrelevance. We have the ability to write the end to this story. The choice is ours.

REFERENCES

1. Fritz C, Curtin J, Poitevineau J, et al. Player preferences among new and old violins. Proc Natl Acad Sci U S A 2012;109(3):760–3.
2. Hounshell D. From the American System to Mass Production, 1800–1932: the development of manufacturing technology in the United States. Detroit (MI): Wayne State University Press; 1984.
3. Ford MR. The lights in the tunnel. United States of America. Acculant Press; 2009.
4. Girard B. The Google way. San Francisco (CA): No Starch Press; 2009.
5. Penenberg AL. Is Google evil? MotherJones.com. 2006. Available at: http://www.motherjones.com/politics/2006/10/google-evil. Accessed June 26, 2012.
6. Aguayo R. Dr. Deming: the American who taught the Japanese about quality. New York: Fireside. 1990.
7. Deming WE. Out of the crisis. Cambridge (United Kingdom): MIT Press; 1986.
8. Ohno T. Toyota production system: beyond large-scale production. New York: Productivity Press; 1988.
9. D'Angelo R, Zarbo RJ. Error reduction and quality management. In: Pantanowitz L, Tuthill JM, Balis U, editors. Pathology informatics: theory and practice. Canada: ASCP Press; 2012. p. 306.
10. Bremner B, Dawson C. Can anything stop Toyota? Businessweek 2003. Available at: http://www.businessweek.com/magazine/content/03_46/b3858001_mz001.htm. Accessed June 20, 2012.
11. Floyd M. Toyota woes continue as Japan launches Prius brakes investigation. MotorTrend 2010. Available at: http://wot.motortrend.com/toyota-woes-continue-as-japan-launches-prius-brakes-investigation-7404.html. Accessed June 21, 2012.
12. Ruffa SA. Going lean: how the best companies apply lean manufacturing principles to shatter uncertainty, drive innovation, and maximize profits. New York: AMACOM; 2008.
13. Antony J. Pros and cons of Six Sigma: an academic perspective. OneSixSigma.com. 2008. Available at: http://web.archive.org/web/20080723015058/http://www.onesixsigma.com/node/7630. Accessed June 22, 2012.
14. Richardson K. The "Six Sigma" factor for Home Depot. Wall Street Journal Online 2007. Available at: http://online.wsj.com/article/SB116787666577566679.html. Accessed June 22, 2012.
15. Google. Google to acquire Motorola mobility. Google Investor Relations 2011. Available at: http://investor.google.com/releases/2011/0815.html. Accessed June 22, 2012.
16. Park S, Pantanowitz L, Parwani AV. Anatomic pathology laboratory information systems: a review. Adv Anat Pathol 2012;19(2):81–96.
17. D'Angelo R, Zarbo RJ. The Henry Ford production system. Am J Clin Pathol 2007; 128:423–9.

18. Aller R, Georgiou A, Pantanowitz L. Electronic health records. In: Pantanowitz L, Tuthill JM, Balis U, editors. Pathology informatics: theory and practice. Canada: ASCP Press; 2012. p. 217–30.

19. Balis U, Pantanowitz L. Specimen tracking and identification systems. In: Pantanowitz L, Tuthill JM, Balis U, editors. Pathology informatics: theory and practice. Canada: ASCP Press; 2012. p. 283–304.

20. Mantha GS, Wiehagen L, Bird J, et al. Implementation of the Toyota Production System in striving for a seamless method to manage patient specimens. Poster session presented at: UPMC Shadyside 2008 Quality and Innovation Fair. Pittsburgh, June 2008.

21. Pantanowitz L, Valenstein PN, Evans AJ, et al. Review of the current state of whole slide imaging in pathology. J Pathol Inform 2011;2:36.

22. Parwani AV, Mojanty SK, Becich MJ. Pathology reporting in the 21st century: the impact of synoptic reports and digital imaging. Lab Med 2008;39:582–6.

23. Pantanowitz L, Hornish M, Goulart R. Informatics applied to cytology. Cytojournal 2008;5:16.

24. Pantanowitz L, Balis U, Parwani AV. Laboratory automation. In: Pantanowitz L, Tuthill JM, Balis U, editors. Pathology informatics: theory and practice. Canada: ASCP Press; 2012. p. 147–55.

25. Middleton SR. Developing an automation concept that is right for your laboratory. Clin Chem 2000;46:757–63.

26. Astles JR, Lubarsky D, Loun B. Pneumatic transport exacerbates interference of room air contamination in blood gas samples. Arch Pathol Lab Med 1996;120:642–7.

27. Felder RA, Savory J, Margrey KS, et al. Development of a robotic near patient testing laboratory. Arch Pathol Lab Med 1995;119:948–51.

28. Pfiefer G. Roadmap to autoverification: simple steps to automate your lab's total manual verification process are provided. Advance Lab 2010;32–6.

29. Dean P. Automation, informatics solutions in clinical chemistry. Advance Lab 2009;35–6.

30. Beck AH, Sangoi AR, Leung S, et al. Systematic analysis of breast cancer morphology uncovers stromal features associated with survival. Sci Transl Med 2011;3(108):108ra113.

31. Le QV, Ranzato MA, Monga R, et al. Building high-level features using large scale unsupervised learning. Presented at the International Conference on Machine Learning. Edinburgh, Scotland, June 25–July 1, 2012.

32. Reis-Filho JS, Weigelt B, Fumagalli D, et al. Molecular profiling: moving away from tumor philately. Sci Transl Med 2010;2(47):47ps43.

33. Henricks WH. "Meaningful use" of electronic health records and its relevance to laboratories and pathologists. J Pathol Inform 2011;2:7.

34. Herper M. The future is now: 23andMe now offers all your genes for $999. Forbes 2011. Available at: http://www.forbes.com/sites/matthewherper/2011/09/27/the-future-is-now-23andme-now-offers-all-your-genes-for-999/. Accessed June 27, 2012.

Pathology Resident and Fellow Education in a Time of Disruptive Technologies

James M. Ziai, MD, Brian R. Smith, MD*

KEYWORDS

- Resident education • Pathology • Laboratory medicine • Molecular genetics
- Informatics • In vivo microscopy • Cell therapy • Telepathology

KEY POINTS

- Resident education in pathology must be modified to accommodate new practice models and technologies, including genomics, informatics, digital pathology, therapeutic pathology, and in vivo microscopy.
- Implementation of a comprehensive genomics and personalized medicine curriculum is currently the most pressing need, while incorporation of digital pathology into training is the area that is currently advancing most rapidly.
- The future role for the practicing pathologist in informatics, in vivo microscopy and therapeutic pathology remains somewhat uncertain but these areas must be included in training if the disciplines are ever to be successfully incorporated into the pathologist's clinical portfolio.
- The need for expanded training in these new areas of pathology and laboratory medicine, while maintaining expertise in traditional areas of the discipline, raises serious questions concerning the future of generalist versus subspecialist pathology practice, the nature of training for pathologist-scientists, and the optimal training and certification approach for the discipline.

Even before the introduction of significant disruptive technologies to the practice of pathology, resident education in the discipline had already experienced fundamental changes starting at the beginning of the 21st century.[1] After a 20-year experiment of adding a credentialing year to all pathology training, the requirement was dropped for the residency class starting in 2002, which effectively moved the curriculum for training in both anatomic pathology (AP) and clinical pathology/laboratory medicine (CP) from 5 years to 4 years and for those training in AP-only or CP-only from 4 years to 3. One consequence of the shortening of core training was a marked increase in the number of residents taking subspecialty fellowships. This was driven in part by the demands of the hiring marketplace but was also made necessary by the explosion

Department of Laboratory Medicine, Yale University School of Medicine, Post Office Box 208035, 333 Cedar Street, New Haven, CT 06520-8035, USA
* Corresponding author.
E-mail address: brian.smith@yale.edu

Clin Lab Med 32 (2012) 623–638
http://dx.doi.org/10.1016/j.cll.2012.07.004   labmed.theclinics.com
0272-2712/12/$ – see front matter © 2012 Elsevier Inc. All rights reserved.

of subspecialty medical knowledge and the rapid introduction and continuing growth and evolution of major game-changing (and therefore fundamentally disruptive) technologies in genetics, informatics, digital pathology, therapeutic pathology, and in vivo diagnostics.[1–8] Residency programs have been forced to wrestle with the need to encompass training in these new areas while preserving nearly all of the traditional components of training. In the words of Lewis Carroll's Red Queen: "... it takes all the running you can do, to keep in the same place. If you want to get somewhere else, you must run at least twice as fast as that!"[9]

Subspecialty fellowship choices are therefore increasingly complex, including

Accreditation Council for Continuing Medical Education (ACGME)-accredited programs with available American Board of Pathology (ABP) certification (blood banking, chemical pathology, cytopathology, dermatopathology, forensic pathology, hematology, medical microbiology, molecular genetic pathology, neuropathology, and pediatric pathology)

ACGME-accredited selective pathology programs without available ABP certification (the most common being general surgical pathology, gastrointestinal/hepatic pathology, gynecologic/perinatal pathology, renal pathology, and bone and soft tissue pathology, but including many others)

ABP certifiable subspecialties in a stage of evolution where there is not yet ACGME accreditation of appropriate fellowship programs (clinical informatics)

Non-ACGME, non-ABP fellowships (often paralleling the selective pathology and ABP menus but also including areas such as immunology and transplantation)[2,10]

Reflecting the surge in new knowledge over the last 10 years, both molecular genetic pathology and clinical informatics have been added to the subspecialty certification menu of the ABP and the number of ACGME-sanctioned selective pathology training programs has increased by more than sixfold over that same time period.[2,11] There are now more fellowship slots than graduating residents.[2] It is estimated that fewer than 10% to 20% of graduating residents apply directly for jobs. The rest go on to seek fellowships, and fully 40% of graduating residents intend to complete more than 1 fellowship.[12] Only rare residents (approximately 5%) state that they are looking for a fellowship, because they cannot find a job[12]; hence these trends reflect a fundamental need for increased and broader training rather than some artifact of a mismatched job market.

These data, then, confirm that the discipline of pathology and laboratory medicine is evolving rapidly. The marketplace for residents/fellows and those hiring them is demanding increasing clinical expertise in the classical pathology subdisciplines as new technologies are introduced into those subdisciplines. Moreover, expertise in these new areas of pathology knowledge is needed to incorporate the disruptive technologies (eg, genomics, digital pathology, informatics) into standard practice. Further reflecting this, and despite the publication of recently updated comprehensive curricula in both AP and CP[13,14] as well as curricula in a number of rapidly growing subspecialty areas,[15–20] the College of American Pathologists and the Association of Pathology Chairs have recognized a critical need to further modify clinical training in an ongoing and dynamic fashion.[21] Finally, since 24% of graduating pathology trainees seek employment in academic medical centers,[12] one must also keep in mind the potential need to alter paradigms for meeting the training requirements of nascent physician–scientists,[22] as well as the training needs of full-time community practitioners.

This article will discuss the effects of the exploding knowledge base on 5 broad areas of resident training that have all been subject to the recent introduction of

disruptive technologies: genomics, digital pathology, in vivo microscopy, informatics, and cell therapy.

GENOMICS EDUCATION

A curriculum for training in genomics and personalized medicine is currently the most critical educational component requiring further development in pathology residency programs. The pace at which the instrumentation and clinical applications of next-generation sequencing (NGS) and whole genome amplification (WGA) technologies develop continues to increase. Thus, pathologists will find themselves increasingly at the center of not only disease testing, result interpretation, and diagnosis, but also preventive medicine, practicing what some have alluded to as primary care pathology.[21] The aim of training residents in the interpretation and management of genetic information, and for an expanding consultative role in clinical medicine, should therefore be paramount in all pathology residency programs.

In 2010, leaders from national pathology organizations and other interest groups gathered at the Banbury Conference at Cold Spring Harbor, New York, to address these issues. They sought to define the anticipated roles pathologists will play in the era of genomic medicine and devised action themes (blue dot projects) to guarantee pathology's future as a discipline (**Box 1**).[23]

By consensus, training future pathologists in genomics and personalized medicine (project 1) is critical to ensuring pathology's place as a vital consultative and clinical service in the postgenomic era. Data[24] show that medical students are primarily taught genetics in the form of a broad survey course early in their training but without significant attention to genomics or its clinical applications or implications.

To this end, Haspel and colleagues[19,25] issued a call to action, proposing and implementing a 5-month curriculum in genomics and personalized medicine at their own institution consisting of resident presentations, lectures, and an optional offering of direct-to-consumer genome sequencing to trainees. The lecture component consists of 4 1-hour lectures focusing on personal genomics, high-throughput sequencing technologies, and genetic counseling in the first month. The first lecture discusses the direct-to-consumer genomic testing experience: specifically, the potential of genomics to improve understanding and management of health and disease, the standards of scientific evidence applied to gene–disease associations, methods of risk

---

Box 1
Banbury Conference blue dot projects for pathology

1. Establish a nationwide pilot program to ensure that every ACGME-approved residency in pathology in North America includes a mandatory curriculum in genomics and personalized medicine.

2. Compile and analyze the full range of current testing offered by pathologists in tissue diagnostics and laboratory medicine and determine which tests might be replaced by NGS or other high-throughput technologies.

3. Establish a clinical grade variant database.

4. Identify and validate operational models for WGA.

5. Formulate regulatory guidelines to conduct whole-genome test accreditation.

6. Define the concept of the primary care pathologist in genome-era medicine.

7. Address reimbursement issues.

assessment, and educational and informational resources for personalized genomics. The second lecture addresses NGS technology and its role(s) in the clinical setting: the limitations of Sanger sequencing, the advantages and disadvantages of different NGS platforms, and how NGS will affect pathology practice. The interpretation of key metrics and parameters that govern an NGS sequencing project is also reviewed. The third lecture discusses genetic counseling. Beginning with an examination of the definition of genetic counseling, the evidence for single nucleotide polymorphism (SNP) associations with disease is analyzed, and residents are instructed in the interpretation of genetic results in the context of other health information. A critical component of the lecture is a discussion of the pathologist's role in interpretation of genetic data (ie, how the consumers' understanding of the health implications of their sequencing results might differ from a health professional's). The ethical implications of sequencing and direct-to-consumer genetic testing are also considered. Finally, methods in literature review and the application of genomic findings to daily practice are presented in the fourth lecture.

In the second and third months, residents are offered the opportunity to send personal samples for exome sequencing. At the same time, they are given a list of risk factors screened for by 3 personalized genomics companies and asked to discuss 1 panel with a faculty member for subsequent presentation in the fifth month. The curriculum closes with discussions regarding the implications of clinical genomics and personalized medicine.

At the time of this initial call to action, few pathology residency programs had active genomics curricula. A survey sent to 185 residency programs in the pathology program directors' section of the Association of Pathology Chairs received 42 responses. Sixty-nine percent of respondents did not have a genomics curriculum in place. Ninety-one per cent of programs without a genomics curriculum desired one. The majority (84%) of these programs planned to implement one: within 3 months (4.3%), 6 months (13%), 1 year (30.4%), or at an indefinite future time (43.5%). However, lack of resident time and limited faculty leaders were the most significant obstacles to implementing a curriculum. Other difficulties may also exist. Haspel and colleagues[25] noted the Stanford experience, in which the debate over personal genetic testing offered to medical students in a medical genetics course led to a moratorium on the option. Proposing the inclusion of optional genetic testing in genomics curricula stems from the idea that the need to know could motivate trainees to more completely assimilate and critically interpret lecture materials and information regarding NGS technology and result interpretation. Haspel and colleagues[25] also noted concerns regarding the necessity of institutional review board (IRB) approval for resident testing as well as possible conflicts of interest with faculty members affiliated with testing companies. In addition to these issues, challenges in training also include the rapidly evolving nature of items 3 through 7 from the Banbury Conference (see **Box 1**) report.[26] For example, the development of a clinical grade human variation database remains in its infancy, although progress is indeed being made.[27–30]

While these are all justifiable concerns, institutions can certainly tailor their approach to genomics education based on resident and faculty consensus. Survey responses from programs without genomics curricula have indicated that access to online lectures and examinations would be the 2 most helpful factors in adopting a genomics curriculum. The public availability of lectures from the Beth Israel-Deaconess (BIDMC) curriculum (genomicmedicineinitiative.org) should facilitate creation of curricula in programs that currently do not have one.[24]

Regardless of how a program structures a genomics curriculum, the objective to train future pathologists as clinical diagnosticians in the analysis and interpretation of genetic data should be central. While understanding NGS technology is important, the rate at which the methodologies change can quickly render any instruction in a particular platform or methodology obsolete. However, practice in the interpretation of sequencing results, in the context of a medical history or other pertinent medical data, is critical to form in residents' minds an idea of their potential role as clinical consultants as well as preparing them to function in this role.

Recently, creation of a third training track in genomic pathology (GP) has been proposed by Musser[31] in anticipation of the increasingly central role that molecular genetic pathologists will play in clinical medicine. Because genomics will undoubtedly affect practice in both surgical pathology and CP, he envisions molecular genetic pathologists playing essential roles in both disciplines, bridging what has in some institutions become a balkanized service. He argues that while the current AP/CP training structure provides exposure to molecular pathology, the field is growing too large and changing too rapidly for residents to be adequately educated in the 1 to 2 months most training programs currently dedicate to it. Relative to the current training system, a GP track could provide the adequate breadth and depth of exposure to molecular genetic pathology necessary to create molecular pathologists competent to practice in the postgenomic era. It is also tempting to further envision opportunities that a GP track might create. As exome and whole genome sequencing become more commonplace, informatics (including storage, mining, and analysis of these data) will become increasingly important in both clinical and research applications. Part of the increased time afforded by a dedicated genomics track could be used for significant statistical and informatics training so molecular pathologists might also serve to bridge the gap between clinical medicine and laboratory informatics, playing vital roles not only in mining and analysis of genomic data to guide clinical care but also possibly the design and implementation of more efficient repositories for these data and their inclusion in the hospital laboratory information system (LIS). Nevertheless, while the development of a full third GP track is certainly one approach that could be taken, it can also be argued that GP will become so integral to all pathology practices that it will be more efficacious to train all pathologists in this subdiscipline, and not just a subset of pathologists. This goal might therefore be best served by integration of genomic training into the existing tracks rather than through creation of a separate track.

Developing methods to assess resident competency in genomics is also critical to a successful curriculum. Competency can be primarily measured in 2 ways: (1) observed performance during rounds, and departmental or interdepartmental presentations, and (2) performance on written or oral examination, such as the Resident In Service Exam (RISE). While genomics questions have been incorporated into RISE examinations with increasing frequency, additional modes of assessment such as presentations and journal club leadership should also be incorporated into programs for several reasons. First, they provide residents with periodic responsibilities that forcibly engage them to learn and present current topics in genomics and molecular pathology. Second, they give the resident further practice in the critical analysis of issues in molecular genetic medicine. Third, these presentations serve as important feedback opportunities to help the resident gauge his or her comfort level and comprehension of topics in genomics. In an ideal world, competency would also be assessed by observation of actual clinical practice. This may remain challenging during the current period while this sort of clinical consultation remains in its infancy and as this role begins to be more broadly accepted as a component of the pathologist's clinical responsibilities.

An equally important component of training residents for practice in the postgenomic era is education in the opportunities and careers involving molecular genetic pathology. Berman and colleagues[30] noted that trainees often elect jobs focused on routine diagnosis since they are unaware of opportunities for pathologists in more molecular-focused research and development arenas, a trend that threatens pathologists' future in guiding patient care, not to mention advancing clinical medicine. It is imperative that residency programs expose and inspire trainees to pursue molecular pathology so that the next generation of pathologists will assume roles as leaders and catalysts in the practice of medicine, rather than relegating themselves to ancillary roles or providing results from just another test. The pathologist's central consultative role must continue to expand in the face of disruptive technologies.

DIGITAL PATHOLOGY AND TELEPATHOLOGY EDUCATION

The terms digital pathology, telepathology, and virtual microscopy have arisen at different times during digital technology's increasing presence in pathology practice, and their definitions have correspondingly evolved. With the advent of whole-slide scanners in 1990, digital pathology initially referred to whole-slide scanning and interpretation. However, as Soenksen has noted,[32] virtual microscopy now better defines this process. A more practical definition of digital pathology now includes not only whole-slide scanning but the entire digital information system from which a pathologist can draw to render a diagnosis. The homepage of the Digital Pathology Association defines it as "a dynamic, image-based environment that enables the acquisition, management and interpretation of pathology information generated from a digitized glass slide."[33]

The benefits of virtual microscopy in medical education have been extensively documented and discussed.[34–39] Harris and colleagues[34] noted increased self-study markedly increased student satisfaction and maintained test performance among medical students in histology laboratory courses using virtual microscopy with annotations and practice exercises. At the resident education level, Web-based slide collections now available containing both static images as well as whole-scanned slides give residents immediate access to a case set of unparalleled breadth including multiple examples of many rare entities (**Table 1**). The annotation of key diagnostic features coupled with ancillary testing images or data including immunohistochemistry, fluorescence in situ hybridization (FISH), or molecular testing results also make such Web sites ideal for self-teaching, since annotation features have been demonstrated to improve comprehension.[34]

One of the most exciting potential applications of virtual microscopy and digital pathology in resident education is in competency assessment. Currently, objective assessments of resident aptitude during training are limited. Bruch and colleagues[35] have designed in-service competency examinations using virtual microscopy to discriminate ability levels among trainees. Scores on this virtual slide examination showed reliability comparable to the discriminating ability of multiple choice questions that are currently more commonly used, as measured by Cronbach's α (0.84), a coefficient of reliability commonly used to demonstrate internal consistency or reliability of a test score. Scores also correlated well with RISE performance. Importantly, the examination was easy to administer and well-accepted by trainees. The use of periodic virtual slide examinations is attractive as a way to objectively measure resident ability and progress throughout training.

Although in-service examinations provide a measure of performance relative to other trainees, these measures do not provide feedback on specific errors in interpretation, analysis or decision-making. Moreover, these tests do not provide guidance on how to arrive at the correct answer, which, in the case of missed morphology or immunohistochemistry questions, make errors in thought or practice difficult to rectify.

Table 1
Some web-based digital slide collections

Web Site	Web Address	Features
California Tumor Tissue Registry	www.cttr.org	Repository of over 30,000 accessions and 30,000 consultations offering subscription-based access to cases, which include clinical history, slide images, diagnosis, and commentary by contributing pathologists
The Rosai Collection	rosaicollection.org	Over 20,000 virtual cases with clinical history summaries, discussions, diagnoses, and commentary by Dr. Juan Rosai and other leading experts
College of American Pathologists–Case of the Month	www.cap.org	Archived monthly surgical pathology unknown cases dating back to 2008, which include clinical history, laboratory findings, virtual slides, and assessment questions
University of Pittsburgh–Surgical Pathology Case of the Month	http://path.upmc.edu/ casemonth/ap-casemonth.html	Archived monthly surgical and clinical pathology unknown cases dating back to 1995, which include clinical history, laboratory findings and slide images with extensive case commentary and analysis
Pathology Outlines	www.pathologyoutlines. com	Surgical and clinical pathology cases organized by topic or organ system with links to images and references; updated regularly
US and Canadian Academy of Pathology–Virtual Slidebox	http://uscap.org/index. htm?vsbindex.htm	Over 450 cases indexed by subspecialty with accompanying virtual slides, immunohistochemistry, and case explanation from renowned contributing pathologists
University of Iowa–Virtual Slide Box	www.path.uiowa.edu/ virtualslidebox	Educational Web site with histology and histopathology atlases in virtual slide form

(*continued on next page*)

Table 1 *(continued)*		
Web Site	**Web Address**	**Features**
Virtual Dermpath	www.virtualdermpath.com	Subscription-based online virtual microscope with quizzes, videos and over 600 virtual slides
Johns Hopkins Surgical Pathology Unknown Conference	pathology2.jhu.edu/sp/	Extensive archived weekly unknown case series with slide and immunohistochemistry images and accompanying case discussion

Practicing pathologists can also make use of these technologies for continuing medical education (CME) requirements. For example, the College of American Pathologists' online virtual biopsy program (VBP) is a virtual microscopy program offered quarterly with 5 diagnostic cases per activity that allows pathologists to evaluate a variety of challenging cases and receive peer review. Each case typically contains a virtual slide, clinical history, diagnostic findings and other ancillary testing data, and sometimes gross, radiographic, or endoscopic findings. Participants receive immediate feedback as they select ancillary studies and diagnoses from a master list, and participants can obtain 5.75 Continuing Medical Education/Self-Assessment Module (CME/SAM) credits after answering 70% or more of the post-test items.

Hamilton and colleagues[36] have taken a more detailed approach to slide interpretation and diagnostic decision making. They have developed a Bayesian Belief Networks-based virtual microscopy model (currently available at www.pathxl.com) to assess morphologic examination practices relative to an expert. The process of examining a slide to arrive at a correct diagnosis is initially modeled by an expert pathologist and then deconstructed into a number of discrete steps. Each step corresponds to observation of a morphologic clue tracked either by eye or slide movement. Each of these steps can then be incorporated into a Bayesian Belief Network system, which calculates the probability of the diagnostic outcome given the observations made. As a trainee examines the slide, the probability of his or her arriving at a correct diagnosis can be estimated in real-time based on his or her movements around the slide. Models such as this provide immediate objective data on case analysis aptitude. They quickly identify errors in decision making while at the same time providing the remedial feedback of a proven structured analysis sequence. Coupled with periodic virtual slide examinations, this approach may provide an indispensable method of not only objectively assessing resident competency and progress but also pinpointing and rectifying errors in diagnostic decision making.

Telepathology has been defined as the practice of pathology at any distance greater than that which allows the pathologist to control the microscope hands on.[38–40] Since its original conception and definition by Weinstein[41] in 1986, telepathology has played only a minor role in daily pathology practice. As Weinstein and colleagues[40] noted, a PubMed search of the term telepathology yields 3 articles before 1990 and 628 by December 2008. Currently, a PubMed search of telepathology yields approximately 800 articles and underscores not only the field's technological advances but also the increasing adoption of telepathology services in both private and academic pathology practices. Laboratory Economics' Digital Pathology Trends Survey conducted in 2010 surveyed 255 academic centers, private practice groups, and commercial laboratories, and found 22% of respondents had existing telepathology facilities, with an additional 20% planning to add facilities within 12 to 24 months.[42] An assessment of the US digital pathology market shows even greater growth, with market values more than doubling between 2004 ($27 million) and 2009 ($60 million) and an average 15% to 20% growth rate since then.[42]

Multiple barriers exist to more widespread use of telepathology in daily practice and include lack of pathology imaging standards, LIS compatibility issues, and cost. And while the largest cited obstacle to more widespread implementation of telepathology services has been cost, the second most frequent reported barrier has been devotion to established methods ("traditional pathology/microscope work fine").[42] Thus, the explicit education of trainees as well as current pathologists in the technology, methods, and practice of telepathology and digital pathology is essential to the further growth of this modality.

INFORMATICS EDUCATION

Pathologists have been urged to recognize informatics as an integral part of their practice for over 20 years.[43–46] Now, in the postgenomic era, this is even more urgent. As whole-exome and whole-genome sequencing become more commonplace in clinical practice, the burden of clinically actionable data will increase almost exponentially, potentially over a time course of decades. Coupled with the increasing centrality of the electronic medical record (EMR) in collating patient data, storage, navigation, and mining of genomic and phenomic data for clinical as well as research purposes will only become more important.[47,48] Pathologists have the potential to establish themselves as key contributors in these endeavors.

Several different approaches have been taken to implementing informatics curricula. Henricks and colleagues[20,49] have proposed goals and objectives for an informatics curriculum including didactic sessions on fundamentals of general computing, laboratory information systems including data standards, and systems management with corresponding exercises for application of knowledge acquired in the didactic sessions. Kang and colleagues[50] have tested a self-directed virtual informatics rotation consisting of 24 recorded lectures, 21 tutorials, and 4 exercises, as well as corresponding textbook readings and online module quizzes. User feedback has been positive, and they report an average 24.3% increase in pretest versus posttest scores.

The data from Kang and colleagues are encouraging and may provide a viable way to speed the adoption of informatics curricula, which has otherwise been slow due to multiple factors including lack of dedicated faculty and time constraints. Regardless of the form a curriculum takes, instruction in informatics should aim to provide didactic and practical instruction in current topics to enable trainees to not only proficiently navigate existing information technologies but also make sound decisions regarding information management and learn and integrate new information beyond the training period. The challenges here are similar to those in the teaching of laboratory management[15] and may be solved through similar approaches.

IN VIVO MICROSCOPY EDUCATION

The revolution in bio-optics has the potential to create another paradigm shift in pathology with the development of miniature microscopes that can be used with endoscopes, vascular catheter-based devices, and other minimally invasive fine needle and other techniques, to allow for point-of-care, real-time, in situ tissue examination with high resolution.[51] Technologies range from optical coherence tomography (OCT) to confocal and other approaches.[52] Resolution is remarkably high, with the major limitation being penetration through only 2 to 3 cell diameters. The technology does not simply potentially replace physical biopsy approaches or allow for directed rather than random biopsies for ex vivo examination but also opens new areas for pathology practice. For example, in examining coronary arteries as well as the central nervous system, the in vivo microscopy approach opens new diagnostic vistas, since physical biopsy is currently impractical or limited in its indications, whereas in vivo microscopy would be more likely to be applied on a routine basis. Although most such medical practice is currently confined to translational research protocols, there is remarkably fast growth in this field of in vivo microscopy (IVM) and rapid extension into clinical practice. As of 2012, over 50 academic medical centers were using IVM clinically and/or developing new technologies in this area, and there were at least 23 vendors developing commercial IVM instruments for the US market with two-thirds based on OCT technology and one-third on confocal technology (Leonard D, Glassy E, Shevchuk M, personal communication, April 15, 2012). The number of publications in the area exceeded 3000 in 2011. Hence, pathology residency programs should be prepared to introduce this technology and clinical approach to their trainees to assure preparation for a likely future.

How the pathologist will interact with this new technology and with nonpathologist clinicians, including radiologists, gastroenterologists, ophthalmologists, cardiologists, and others, remains undefined.[53,54] A College of American Pathologists survey in 2010 determined that only 34% of pathologists were familiar with IVM, and only 2% had any direct experience; only 12% expected to be involved directly in IVM over the succeeding 5 years.[54] This, of course, combined with the existence of appropriate infrastructure at only a few medical centers, makes it difficult to determine how best to introduce residents to this technology. Nevertheless, the authors believe that the game-changing nature of this new clinical approach makes it imperative that training programs begin to plan for its incorporation into the educational program, potentially in concert with radiology, gastroenterology, and other medical colleagues.

THERAPEUTIC PATHOLOGY EDUCATION

The pathology community has consistently thought of its role in the care of the patient as the diagnostic specialty, and indeed the vast majority of the pathologist's current workload is clearly in that arena. All of the prior disruptive technologies discussed also aim predominantly in that direction. For example, the role of the pathologist in in vivo microscopy is thought of as diagnosing the lesion but is certainly not considered by the vast majority of pathologists to also include performing a minimally invasive treatment of the disease once diagnosed. Some have suggested expanding the pathologist's diagnostic role by envisioning a future department of diagnostics that involves imaging (radiology) as well as pathology and laboratory medicine activities.[55] Despite the appearance of such a fictional department on the popular television show "House," however, it seems unlikely that this sort of medical reorganization will occur anytime soon.[56]

Yet an alternative view of the discipline of pathology would not limit the pathologist's role based on whether an activity is diagnostic or therapeutic but rather whether or not the activity uses the clinical laboratory, regardless of whether the goal of the laboratory's activity is diagnostic or therapeutic.[7] Such an approach would represent, in some respects, a simple expansion of the pathologist's current role in transfusion medicine, in particular, to include all laboratory aspects of the rapidly emerging field of regenerative medicine.[57,58] These therapies represent yet another arm of personalized medicine: manipulating autologous cells in the laboratory for immunotherapy against cancer, creation of new vasculature for cardiopulmonary disease and other uses of progenitor cells, and manipulation of the immune system in the case of infectious and autoimmune disorders, as well as the potential for individualized vaccine and protein therapeutics. Currently, translational cell therapy protocols most frequently involve preparation of the personalized therapy by an in-house good manufacturing practices (GMP) facility.[59,60] There are many advantages to this localized approach but also many challenges, as such therapies move toward standard of care and hence roll out to smaller medical centers. An alternative future model might therefore be that of centralized facilities that may operate independent of pathologists, a model that has been used for the US Food and Drug Administration (FDA)-approved autologous T-cell therapy for metastatic castrate-resistant prostate cancer (Sipuleucel-T, Provenge).[61] How the infrastructure of the future will look for regenerative medicine technologies remains unknown. Moreover, as in the case of IVM and other disruptive technologies, it remains unclear whether pathologists will embrace this extension of their current activities or cede the area of cellular therapy to other disciplines.

If pathology does embrace this therapeutic subdiscipline, then there is a real need for thoughtful and comprehensive educational and competency assessment approaches for residents. Interestingly, although thought has been given to educating physicians in the delivery of such cellular biologics, especially in cardiovascular medicine,[62] relatively little has been written concerning specific education in the actual on-site production of stem cell and progenitor, immunocyte, or personalized vaccine therapeutics, although recent transfusion medicine curricula have outlined a very reasonable approach for training pathology residents in this area.[16,63–65] Perhaps the question is not whether residents need to be trained in therapeutic pathology, but rather when.

EDUCATING THE PHYSICIAN–SCIENTIST

Pathology is a major haven for the physician–scientist career pathway. Students from Medical Scientist Training Program (MSTP) MD/PhD programs choose internal medicine as their most popular career choice but pathology as their second most popular choice.[22,66] Moreover, of all the disciplines that MD/PhD students choose, those who go into pathology have the lowest likelihood of entering full-time private clinical practice.[67] Hence this is a committed group of trainees that should not be lost sight of as the best educational approaches are planned for the next generation of pathologists.

In internal medicine, pediatrics, and several other disciplines, specific educational and residency/fellowship training pathways are endorsed and promulgated by their respective national board and residency review committee organizations.[68,69] These pathways combine curriculum requirements specific to this career choice, allow for integrated longitudinal experiences in research and clinical activities, and generally compress some elective clinical training in favor of increased research exposure. Pathology has not chosen this route, but instead has favored development of such programs by individual institutions, which are therefore not constrained by a single national consensus approach. Whether the individualized institutional approach versus a national standards approach is best for the discipline and the trainees can be argued, but regardless of which approach is used, it is clear that 1 of the challenges for the future education of pathologist–scientists will be combining the increasing time demands of a rigorous research preparatory pathway with the increasing clinical demands of an ever-expanding discipline, especially if all of the disruptive technologies noted above come to pass as part of a pathologist's armamentarium.

The case of the pathologist–scientist, therefore, highlights a more general question and concern for training, that is, how to expand the clinical reach of the entire pathology profession, which is being driven to expand by the advent of disruptive technologies, while at the same time maintaining core competency in all areas of practice by individual pathologists. Indeed, this is a question that has been faced by all major medical disciplines in an era of rapidly expanding biomedical knowledge. In pathology, can one continue with only minor tweaks to residency and fellowship training, or will there be a time when more radical approaches to the global delivery of pathology services by individual pathologists must be contemplated?

SHOULD THERE BE MULTIPLE CAREER PATHWAYS IN PATHOLOGY?

Given the increasing complexity of potential future pathology practice, the question arises as to whether pathology will remain with its current clinical model, where the typical pathologist performs all tasks in the broad continuum of AP and CP, plus, in the near future, all the new demands outlined in this article, or whether, like most other medical disciplines, pathology must move toward a more subspecialty model of practice. In some respects, the move toward subspecialization is already in full swing, as residents and practices vote with their feet by demanding more and more subspecialty training. This trend, however, remains constrained by virtue of the unique topography of pathology practice. Whereas a hematologist–oncologist or nephrologist or thoracic surgeon may easily have enough patient encounters within a 15-mile radius of his or her primary office location to justify a busy subspecialty practice, it is less likely that a full-time hematopathologist or transfusion medicine specialist, or renal pathologist would be in a similar situation. However, as medical care delivery models move toward larger and larger practice units with better and better electronic transfer of medical information, and as telepathology expands, it may become more realistic for pathology practices to include a majority of their members as subspecialists. As in areas like internal medicine/hematology, where full-time practice in this 1 subspecialty is generally not realistic, and hence most physicians in that discipline practice hematology together with medical oncology, pathologists may do the same, combining 2 or more pathology subdisciplines. Since 40% of residents currently plan on 2 or more fellowships, market pressures are already clearly moving in this direction. If this becomes the definitive trend, is it time to consider a pathology training model that more explicitly produces subspecialists rather than generalists?

These issues bring to the forefront certain questions that must be answered by the pathology community. If the current residency model holds, how will pathology include training in the new areas outlined in this article and still maintain the current timeline for training? Is it realistic to include training in genomics consultation, informatics, IVM, and therapeutic pathology in addition to an already exploding base of knowledge in classical AP and CP, without increasing time for training or moving to a revised paradigm of subspecialty practice? It seems clear that to add much more content will require subtracting something else, but what? Some have argued that it is time to add another year or perhaps even multiple years of training in core pathology, but even if there were more time for initial training, how does one deal with the need for lifelong learning in such a broadened specialty? These are questions with which the College of American Pathologists, the Association of Pathology Chairs, and many other pathology organizations are beginning to wrestle.[21]

In the turmoil of today's overall health care environment, it has become common to recognize that there are frequently more questions than there are answers. Perhaps all one can be sure of is that pathology training by the middle of the 21st century will likely be radically different from what is seen today.

REFERENCES

1. Alexander CB. Pathology graduate medical education (overview from 2006-2010). Hum Pathol 2011;42(6):763–9.
2. Crawford JM, Hoffman RD, Black-Schaffer WS. Pathology subspecialty fellowship application reform 2007 to 2010. Hum Pathol 2011;42(6):774–94.
3. Myers JL, Yousem SA, DeYoung BR, et al, on behalf of the Council of the Association of Directors of Anatomic and Surgical Pathology. Matching residents to pathology fellowships: the road less traveled? Am J Clin Pathol 2011;135:335–7.
4. Lagwinski N, Hunt JL. Fellowship trends of pathology residents. Arch Pathol Lab Med 2009;133(9):1431–6.
5. Kass ME, Crawford JM, Bennett B, et al, Future of Pathology Task Group. Adequacy of pathology resident training for employment: a survey report from the Future of Pathology Task Group. Arch Pathol Lab Med 2007;131(4):545–55.
6. The case for change. In: Transforming pathologists by CAP. 2012. Available at: http://www.cap.org/apps/docs/membership/transformation/new/transform_index.html. Accessed March 25, 2012.
7. Smith BR. Therapeutic pathology: time to move beyond diagnostics. Hum Pathol 2008;39:1725–7.
8. Scott MG, Smith BR, Wu AHB, et al. How well are we training the next generation of clinical pathologists and clinical laboratory directors? A global perspective. Clin Chem 2012;58:491–5.
9. Carroll L, Gardner M, Tenniel J. Through the looking glass. In: The annotated Alice: the definitive edition. New York: WW Norton; 1999. p. 60.
10. BMS announces certification in two new physician subspecialties: clinical informatics and brain injury medicine. In: ABMS. 2012. Available at: http://www.abms.org/News_and_Events/Media_Newsroom/Releases/release_Announcing_TwoNew Subspecialties_10312011.aspx. Accessed March 23, 2012.
11. Sobel ME, Bagg A, Caliendo AM, et al. The evolution of molecular genetic pathology. J Mol Diagn 2008;10(6):480–3.
12. Rinder HM, Wagner J. ASCP Fellowship & job market surveys: a report on the RISE, FISE, FISHE, and TMISE Surveys. 2011. Available at: http://www.ascp.org/PDF/Fellowship-Reports/2011-ASCP-Fellowship-Job-Market-Surveys.pdf. Accessed March 25, 2012.
13. Smith BR, Wells A, Alexander CB, et al, for the Academy of Clinical Laboratory Physicians and Scientists. Curriculum content and evaluation of resident competency in clinical pathology (laboratory medicine): a proposal. Am J Clin Pathol 2006;125(Suppl 1):S5–7.
14. Association of Directors of Anatomic and Surgical Pathology (ADASP). Curriculum content and evaluation of resident competency in anatomic pathology: a proposal. Am J Clin Pathol 2003;120:652–60.
15. Weiss RL, McKenna BJ, Lord-Toof M, et al, Work Group members. A consensus curriculum for laboratory management training for pathology residents. Am J Clin Pathol 2011;136(5):671–8.
16. Fung MK, Crookston KP, Wehrli G, et al, Taskforce on Transfusion Medicine Resident Curriculum, American Association of Blood Banks. A proposal for curriculum content in transfusion medicine and blood banking education in pathology residency programs. Transfusion 2007;47(10):1930–6.
17. Yu GH, Accreditation Council for Graduate Medical Education. Goals and guidelines for residency training in cytopathology. Diagn Cytopathol 2011;39(6):455–60.

18. Otte KK, Zehe SC, Wood AJ, et al. Legal aspects of laboratory medicine and pathology for residents and fellows: a curriculum for pathology training programs. Arch Pathol Lab Med 2010;134(7):1029–32.

19. Haspel RL, Arnaout R, Briere LA, et al. A call to action: training pathology residents in genomics and personalized medicine. Am J Clin Pathol 2010;133(6):832–4.

20. Henricks WH, Boyer PJ, Harrison JH, et al. Informatics training in pathology residency programs: proposed learning objectives and skill sets for the new millennium. Arch Pathol Lab Med 2013;127(8):1009–18.

21. Talbert ML, Ashwood ER, Brownlee NA, et al. Resident preparation for practice: a white paper from the College of American Pathologists and Association of Pathology Chairs. Arch Pathol Lab Med 2009;133(7):1139–47.

22. Schafer AI, editor. The vanishing physician–scientist? London: Cornell University Press; 2009.

23. Tonellato PJ, Crawford JM, Boguski MS, et al. A national agenda for the future of pathology in personalized medicine. Report of the proceedings of a meeting at the Banbury Conference Center on genome-era pathology, precision diagnostics and preemptive care: a stakeholder summit. Am J Clin Pathol 2011;135:668–72.

24. Haspel RL. What you don't know can hurt you. 2011. Available at: http://lpm.hms.harvard.edu/palaver/sites/default/files/11_04_04_Richard%20Haspel_BMI_714.pdf. Accessed May 2, 2012.

25. Haspel RL, Arnaout R, Briere L, et al. Online supplement: a curriculum in genomics and personalized medicine for pathology residents. Am J Clin Pathol 2010;133. Available at: http://108.167.136.110/~gmi2010/AJCP-June-Supplement.pdf. Accessed May 2 , 2012.

26. Cagle PT, Dacic S, Allen TC. Genomic pathology: challenges for implementation. Arch Pathol Lab Med 2011;135(8):967–8.

27. ISCA consortium partners with sequencing group to develop clinical-grade human variation database. In: Genomeweb, BioArray News. 2012. Available at: http://www.genomeweb.com/arrays/isca-consortium-partners-sequencing-group-develop-clinical-grade-human-variation. Accessed April 16, 2012.

28. Li MJ, Wang P, Liu X, et al. GWASdb: a database for human genetic variants identified by genome-wide association studies. Nucleic Acids Res 2012;40:D1047–54.

29. US Dept. of Health and Human Services. NCBI launches the Database of Genomic Structural Variations. 2010. Available at: http://www.nih.gov/news/health/sep2010/nlm-30.htm. Accessed April 16, 2012.

30. Berman DM, Bosenberg MW, Orwant RL, et al. Investigative pathology: leading the postgenomic revolution. Laboratory Investigation 2012;92:4–8.

31. Musser JM. Third track pathology: in unambiguous support of the Banbury Conference report. Arch Pathol Lab Med 2011;135:687–8.

32. Soenksen D. Digging their way in: digital pathology systems. CAP Today; 2008. p. 70.

33. Digital Pathology Association. Available at: http://digitalpathologyassociation.org/. Accessed April 26, 2012.

34. Harris T, Leaven T, Heidger P, et al. Comparison of a virtual microscope laboratory to a regular microscope laboratory for teaching histology. Anat Rec 2001;265(1):10–4.

35. Bruch LA, De Young BR, Kreiter CD, et al. Competency assessment of residents in surgical pathology using virtual microscopy. Hum Pathol 2009;40:1122–8.

36. Hamilton PW, Wang Y, McCullough SJ. Virtual microscopy and digital pathology in training and education. APMIS 2012;120:305–15.

37. Pantanowitz L, Valenstein PN, Evan AJ, et al. Review of the current state of whole slide imaging in pathology. J Pathol Inform 2011;2(36):1–17.

38. Dee FR. Virtual microscopy in pathology education. Hum Pathol 2009;40: 1112–21.
39. Kayser K, Ogilvie R, Borkenfeld S, et al. E-education in pathology certification of e-institutions. Diag Pathol 2011;6(S11):4.
40. Weinstein RS, Graham AR, Richter LC, et al. Overview of telepathology, virtual microscopy, and whole slide imaging: prospects for the future. Hum Pathol 2009;40(8):1057–69.
41. Weinstein RS. Prospects for telepathology. Hum Pathol 1986;17(5):433–4.
42. Friedman B. Digital pathology adoption trends by pathologists. In: The daily scan following a survey article in Laboratory Economics. 2010. Available at: http://blog. aperio.com/2010/06/index.html. Accessed April 23, 2012.
43. Weinstein RS, Bloom KJ. The pathologist as information specialist [editorial]. Hum Pathol 1990;21:4–5.
44. Harrison JH. Pathology informatics questions and answers from the University of Pittsburgh pathology residency informatics rotation. Arch Pathol Lab Med 2004; 128:71–83.
45. Pantanowitz L, Henricks WH, Beckh BA. Medical laboratory informatics. Clin Lab Med 2007;27:823–43.
46. Park SL, Pantanowitz L, Sharma G, et al. Anatomic pathology laboratory informa- tion systems: a review. Adv Anat Pathol 2012;19(2):81–96.
47. Shublaq NW, Coveney PV. Merging genomic and phenomic data for research and clinical impact. Stud Health Technol Inform 2012;174:111–5.
48. Gabril MY, Yousef GM. Informatics for practicing anatomical pathologists: marking a new era in pathology practice. Mod Pathol 2010;23:349–58.
49. Henricks WH, Healy JC. Informatics training in pathology residency programs. Am J Clin Pathol 2002;118:172–8.
50. Kang HP, Hagenkord JM, Monzon FA, et al. Residency training in pathology infor- matics: a virtual rotation solution. Am J Clin Pathol 2009;132:404–8.
51. Liu JT, Loewke NO, Mandella MJ, et al. Point-of-care pathology with miniature microscopes. Anal Cell Pathol 2011;34(3):81–98.
52. Holmes J. OCT technology development: where are we now? A commercial perspective. J Biophotonics 2009;2:347–52.
53. Turner JW, Baehner FL, Bloom KJ, et al, Technology Assessment Committee (TAC) with input from the Council on Scientific Affairs. In vivo Microscopy. In: CAP.org POET reports. 2010. Available at: http://www.cap.org/apps/cap.portal? _nfpb=true&cntvwrPtlt_actionOverride=%2Fportlets%2FcontentViewer%2Fshow&_ windowLabel=cntvwrPtlt&cntvwrPtlt{actionForm.contentReference}=committees %2Ftechnology%2Fin_vivo.html&_state=maximized&_pageLabel=cntvwr. Acc- essed March 24, 2012.
54. Wallace MB. The changing paradigm of endoscopy and pathology. Available at: http://www.gastro.org/journals-publications/aga-perspectives/august-september- 2010/the-changing-paradigm-of-endoscopy-and-pathology. Accessed April 16, 2012.
55. Ford A. A molecular summit, mix and match diagnostics. In: CAP.org 2008. Available at: http://www.cap.org/apps/cap.portal?_nfpb=true&cntvwrPtlt_actionOverride=% 2Fportlets%2FcontentViewer%2Fshow&_windowLabel=cntvwrPtlt&cntvwrPtlt {actionForm.contentReference}=cap_today%2Ffeature_stories%2F0108_Molecular_ Summit.html&_state=maximized&_pageLabel=cntvwr. Accessed March 25, 2012.
56. Jauhar S. Commentary: magical medicine on TV. New York Times, July 19, 2005. Avail- able at: http://www.nytimes.com/2005/07/19/health/19comm.html. Accessed May 2, 2012.

57. Power C, Rasko JE. Promises and challenges of stem cell research for regenerative medicine. Ann Intern Med 2011;155(10):706–13 W217.

58. Reed W, Noga SJ, Gee AP, et al. Production Assistance for Cellular Therapies (PACT): four-year experience from the United States National Heart, Lung, and Blood Institute (NHLBI) contract research program in cell and tissue therapies. Transfusion 2009;49(4):786–96.

59. Rebulla P, Giordano R. Role of the blood service in cellular therapy. Biologicals 2012;13:282–9.

60. Macpherson JL, Rasko JE. Cellular therapy in the Asia–Pacific region. A guide for the future pathologist. Pathology 2011;43(6):616–26.

61. Di Lorenzo G, Buonerba C, Kantoff PW. Immunotherapy for the treatment of prostate cancer. Nat Rev Clin Oncol 2011;8(9):551–61.

62. Dib N, Menasche P, Bartunek JJ, International Society for Cardiovascular Translational Research. Recommendations for successful training on methods of delivery of biologics for cardiac regeneration: a report of the International Society for Cardiovascular Translational Research. JACC Cardiovasc Interv 2010;3(3): 265–75.

63. Haspel RL. Implementation and assessment of a resident curriculum in evidence-based transfusion medicine. Arch Pathol Lab Med 2010;134(7):1054–9.

64. Sanchez R, Sloan SR, Josephson CD, et al. Consensus recommendations of pediatric transfusion medicine objectives for clinical pathology residency training programs. Transfusion 2010;50(5):1071–8.

65. Wu YY, Tormey C, Stack G. Resident and fellow training in transfusion medicine. Clin Lab Med 2007;27:293–342.

66. Paik JC, Howard G, Lorenz RG. Postgraduate choices of graduates from medical scientist training programs, 2004-2008. JAMA 2009;302:1271–3.

67. Brass LF, Akabas MH, Burnley LD, et al. Are MD-PhD programs meeting their goals? An analysis of career choices made by graduates of 24 MD-PhD programs. Acad Med 2010;85:692.

68. American Board of Internal Medicine Research Pathway policies and requirements. Available at: http://www.abim.org/certification/policies/research-pathway-policies-requirements.aspx. Accessed April 16, 2012.

69. American Board of Pediatrics Integrated Research Pathway. Available at: https://www.abp.org/abpwebsite/becomecert/generalpediatrics/nonstandardpathways/integratedresearch.htm. Accessed April 16, 2012.

Twenty-First Century Pathology Sign-Out

Scott Tomlins, MD, PhD[a], Daniel Robinson, PhD[a],
Robert J. Penny, MD, PhD[b,c], Jay L. Hess, MD, PhD, MHSA[b,*]

KEYWORDS

- Personalized medicine • Molecular diagnostics • Future of pathology

KEY POINTS

- The field of pathology is changing rapidly.
- Molecular diagnostics will complement morphologic diagnosis, directing patients to more specific and effective therapy.
- Changes in technology, data reporting, and new business models will be required for pathologists to continue to play a central role in this age of personalized medicine.

MOVING FROM A GENE TO A PATHWAY PERSPECTIVE IN DIAGNOSIS OF DISEASES

The pace of scientific discovery is nothing short of extraordinary. Not only is there an increasing number of diagnostic category diseases being recognized but also a dramatic expansion of ancillary testing with many implications for therapy and prognosis. Technologies such as high throughput sequencing, for example, have provided numerous insights into tumor biology, but the challenge of transforming the data into actionable results is daunting. The initial optimism that most tumors would be similar to chronic myelogenous leukemia, which is defined by a single molecular abnormality (ie, the BCR-ABL fusion protein), and would respond dramatically to targeted therapy is fading. Instead, most common solid tumors and hematologic malignancies involve a genetic patchwork quilt of abnormalities, some shared between different tumor types but in most cases occurring at low frequencies in any given tumor type. As one example, scientists at the Michigan Center for Translational Pathology, led by Dr Arul Chinnaiyan, recently sequenced the exomes of 50 fatal castrate-resistant prostate cancers (CRPCs) obtained at rapid autopsy (including 3 different foci from the same patient) and 11 treatment-naïve, high-grade localized prostate cancers.[1] In

[a] Department of Pathology, Michigan Center for Translational Pathology, University of Michigan Medical School, 5316 CCGC 0940, 1400 E. Medical Center Drive, Ann Arbor, MI 48109-0940, USA; [b] Department of Pathology, University of Michigan Medical School, 5240 Medical Science 1, 1301 Catherine Street, Ann Arbor, MI 48109-5602, USA; [c] International Genomics Consortium, 445 N. 5th Street, Phoenix, AZ 85004, USA
* Corresponding author.
E-mail address: jayhess@umich.edu

Clin Lab Med 32 (2012) 639–650
http://dx.doi.org/10.1016/j.cll.2012.07.002
0272-2712/12/$ – see front matter © 2012 Elsevier Inc. All rights reserved.

labmed.theclinics.com

combination with previous studies comprehensively profiling gene expression alterations,[1–3] gene fusions,[4,5] noncoding transcripts,[6] copy number changes,[1,2] and structural alterations and mutations,[7] these studies collectively showed a remarkable array of more than 100 potentially pathogenetic molecular abnormalities (**Fig. 1**). Although this work was enormously complex, one of the key findings was that many of the tumors showed abnormalities in a limited set of largely mutually exclusive oncogenes including the *ETS* family translocations, mutations in *RAF/RAS* kinase pathways, and overexpression of *SPINK1*. Against this backdrop of likely driver mutations, several other alterations were seen in specific pathways including androgen signaling, histone modifiers, *PTEN,* and others in advanced and high-grade localized prostate cancers. The number of alterations in histone-modifying proteins was particularly striking. In an increasingly common theme in cancer, mutations are often seen in related family members (eg, *ASXL1, ASXL2, ASXL3*) and members of the same biochemical complex (eg, *DPY30, WDR5, ASH2L, RBBP5, MEN1, MLL2, 3,* and *5*), as well as transcription factors (eg, *FOXA1, ERG*), all of which converge on a common final pathway (in this case, androgen receptor signaling) (**Fig. 2**). Clearly, future pathology reporting, to be comprehensible, will need to take more of a pathway perspective to identify "nodes" that are amenable to a particular type of therapy. Although molecular testing has not played a major role in the management of prostate cancer, it is likely that therapy will be increasingly guided by this type of approach. For example, 1 patient with CRPC in the study cited[1] harbored a somatic, homozygous deletion of *BRCA2* associated with an outlier number of mutations consistent with disruption of DNA repair, suggesting potential therapeutic benefit with a poly(ADP-ribose) polymerase family (PARP) inhibitor.[8] Another patient with CRPC showed a focal, high-level copy gain of cyclin-dependent kinase 4 (CDK4), suggesting potential therapeutic benefit with CDK4 inhibitors (**Fig. 3**).[9] Many patients with CRPC show reactivation of the androgen receptor signaling pathway, suggesting that these would respond to anti–androgen receptor signaling therapy.[10,11] Indeed, exome sequencing identified mutations and/or focal high-level copy gain at the androgen receptor (*AR*) locus in 30 (63%) of 48 CRPCs but 0 of 11 high-grade localized prostate cancers.[1] However, through combined genomic and transcriptomic interrogation, 17 (81%) of 21 CRPCs with androgen-driven *TMPRSS2:ERG* gene fusions retained marked overexpression of *ERG,*[1] providing direct evidence for ongoing androgen signaling. In the future, interrogation of *AR* genomic status (ie, mutation or amplification) and detection of mutations in the entire AR signaling program (including expression of androgen-driven gene fusions), will likely drive the decision of whether to treat with an antiandrogen therapy. In addition, repeat biopsy of the progressing lesions or alternative ways of interrogating lesions after treatment (eg, through circulating tumor cells[12]) may be needed after treatment. Comprehensive molecular analysis has the promise to identify mutations in genes across entire pathways, which could be used to stratify patients toward more general pathway–specific therapies. For example, mutation or high-level copy gain/loss in phosphatase and tenin homolog (*PTEN*) or phosphoinositide-3-kinase, catalytic, alpha peptide (PIK3CA) was identified in 24 (50%) of 48 CRPCs. A pathway-based analysis identified aberrations among PTEN interaction network members in 80% of CRPCs,[1] which may influence the activity of phosphoinositide 3-kinase (PI3K) signaling pathway inhibitors.[13] Two CPRCs showed mutations in *RET* (ie, R873W and R600Q). *RET* harbors recurrent activating mutations in medullary thyroid carcinoma centered on residues close to those observed in prostate cancer (ie, C634, A883, M918), with mutations in R600 having been reported in familial medullary thyroid carcinoma,[14] and a small fraction of lung cancers have been shown to harbor driving gene fusions involving *RET*.[15] Importantly, kinase

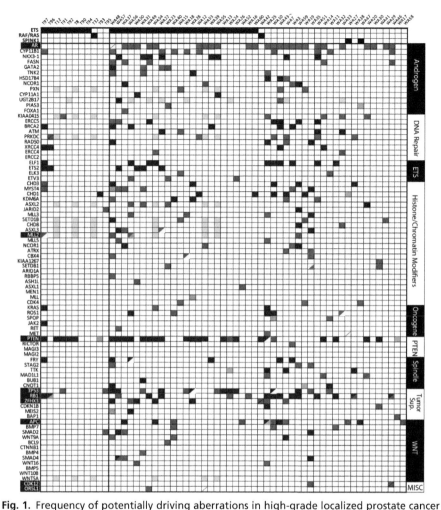

Fig. 1. Frequency of potentially driving aberrations in high-grade localized prostate cancer and lethal metastatic CRPC. An integrated mutational landscape of prostate cancer was identified by sequencing the exomes of 50 CRPCs (WA3–WA60) and 11 high-grade untreated localized prostate cancers (T8–T97).[1] A heatmap of high-level copy number alterations and nonsynonymous mutations is used to visualize potentially driving aberrations. Samples are stratified by localized prostate cancers and CRPCs, *ETS* status, and then ordered by the total number of aberrations in shown genes. *ETS* gene fusions, *RAF/RAS* family aberrations, and *SPINK1* outlier expression are indicated for all samples (black is present). For each gene, aberrations as indicated by the legend are shown (2 aberrations in the same gene are indicated by divided boxes). Blue indicates high-level copy loss; red, high-level copy gain; gray, gene not assessed; yellow, point mutation; orange, frame preserving indel; green, splice-site mutation; and purple, nonsense or frame-shift mutation. Genes identified as significantly mutated across the entire cohort have names in white. (*From* Grasso CS, Wu YM, Robinson DR, et al. The mutational landscape of lethal castrate resistant prostate cancer. Nature 2012;487(7406):239–43; with permission.)

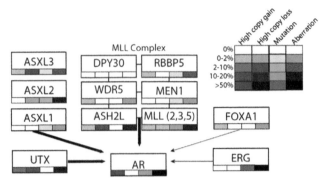

Fig. 2. Example of mutations in elements of androgen signaling pathway. Sequencing exomes of CRPC and high-grade localized prostate cancers identified mutations in several genes that interact with the androgen receptor. The frequency of high copy number alterations, somatic mutations, and both aberration types are shown for chromatin/histone modifiers, the androgen receptor collaborating factor *FOXA1*, and *ERG*, according to the color scales. *MLL* aberration frequency includes *MLL*, *MLL2*, *MLL3,* and *MLL5*. Genes encoding androgen receptor interactors identified by Grasso and colleagues[1] are indicated by bold arrows. (*From* Grasso CS, Wu YM, Robinson DR, et al. The mutational landscape of lethal castrate resistant prostate cancer. Nature 2012;487(7406):239–43; with permission.)

inhibitors such as vandetanib and others show clinical activity in thyroid cancer[16] and preclinical activity in lung cancer models.[15] Finding previously unrecognized *RET* mutations in prostate cancer raises the question of whether targeting of these mutations in CPRC would be effective and what level of evidence would justify taking this approach. One of the goals of the Michigan Oncology Sequencing Project is to address this kind of question—to assess the clinical utility of genomewide sequencing

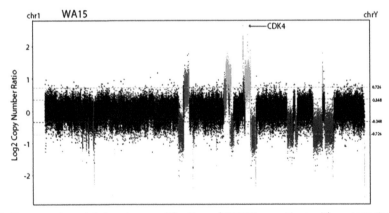

Fig. 3. Copy number plot showing amplification of CDK4 in a patient with metastatic CRPC. Exome sequencing data were used to derive genomewide copy number profiles for CRPCs and localized prostate cancers.[1] The log2 copy number ratio (tumor to normal) for each targeted exon in a patient with CRPC (WA15), ordered by genomic location, is shown. Genes with 1 copy gain/loss are indicated by red and blue points, respectively, and those with >1 copy gain/loss are indicated by orange and cyan points, respectively. The location of a focal amplification including *CDK4* on chr12 is indicated. (*From* Grasso CS, Wu YM, Robinson DR, et al. The mutational landscape of lethal castrate resistant prostate cancer. Nature 2012;487(7406):239–43; with permission.)

and whether enrolling patients with cancer in clinical trials of such targeted therapies is warranted (**Fig. 4**).[17] In this institutional review board–approved research study, patients with advanced cancer underwent repeat biopsy and their DNA and RNA samples from the tumor, along with DNA from healthy tissue, is comprehensively analyzed for translocations, mutations, deletions, additions, and RNA expression levels. Bioinformatic analysis typically reveals more than 100 mutations and other abnormalities in a given tumor. The sequencing results are reviewed at interdisciplinary tumor boards involving pathologists, oncologists, bioinformatics scientists, clinical genetic counselors, and bioethicists. Therapeutic hypotheses are developed and particular abnormalities further confirmed by Sanger sequencing before enrolling patients in particular clinical trials of drugs to which they are predicted to have a higher likelihood of responding. One of the themes that is emerging from this and other studies, such as the prostate cancer study discussed earlier, is that the same cellular pathways are altered in a wide range of tumors. This is significant because of the plethora of new agents that are available that target specific pathways. For example, the anaplastic lymphoma kinase is activated via translocation in almost all cases of anaplastic large cell lymphoma and via different translocation in 5% of non–small cell lung cancer cases and is mutated in 5% to 10% of neuroblastoma cases. All of these tumor types are responsive to the anaplastic lymphoma kinase inhibitor crizotinib.

NEW STRATEGIES ARE NEEDED FOR TRANSLATING MOLECULAR DATA INTO ACTIONABLE RESULTS

With the increasing number of potential molecular abnormalities, the approach of testing for individual mutations is becoming less and less feasible. With the cost of genomewide next-generation sequencing falling dramatically and with shorter

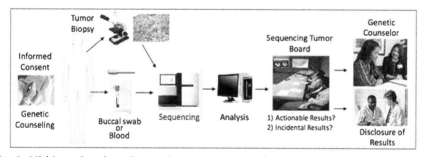

Fig. 4. Michigan Oncology Sequencing Project: an exploratory integrative sequencing of tumors study for personalized oncology. The Michigan Oncology Sequencing Project, instituted at the Michigan Center for Translational Pathology, is a novel approach to personalized oncology. Patients are provided upfront genetic counseling, and patients are tracked through a biospecimen and clinical database. Whole-genome sequencing, whole-exome sequencing, and transcriptome sequencing are performed on tumor specimens to comprehensively identify structural rearrangements, copy number alterations, point mutations, and aberrant gene expression. Results are analyzed at multidisciplinary sequencing tumor boards that include experts in clinical oncology, genomics, bioinformatics, pathology, bioethics, and genetics. Results are reported back to the referring clinician in a clinically relevant time frame (≤3 weeks). (*Adapted from* Roychowdhury S, Iyer MK, Robinson DR, et al. Personalized oncology through integrative high-throughput sequencing: a pilot study. Sci Transl Med 2011;3(111):111–21; with permission.)

instrument run times, sequencing-based diagnosis is rapidly becoming a clinical reality. Although this represents an exciting future, formidable challenges lie ahead. The process of selecting therapeutic targets at present is challenging. The frequency of mutations in different tumor types offers some clues as to what are driver, as opposed to passenger, mutations, but this process of discernment is in its infancy. Several different inputs are likely to go into the pathology reports of the future to make them more clinically useful (**Fig. 5**). *Tumor Genomics* using data sources such as The Cancer Genome Atlas project can provide information on how frequently a given mutation occurs in 20 common human cancers, with the general strategy that recurrent abnormalities would be expected to have a higher likelihood of being tumor-driving mutations compared with isolated mutations. *Model System Genomics* is a related strategy that takes advantage of databases reporting sequencing and copy number variations in panels of cell lines such as the Welcome Trust Sanger Institute Cancer Cell Line Project (785 cell lines), GlaxoSmithKline/caBIG GSK300 Project (300 cell lines), and Broad-Novartis Cancer Cell Line Encyclopedia (886 cell lines). Just as in primary tumors, recurrent mutations point to genes that are more likely to have driver mutations. Another strategy is to use information gleaned from *Functional Genomics* screens. In these types of experiments, panels of tumor cell lines are targeted by large libraries of small interfering RNAs or short hairpin RNAs to block expression and then make inferences on which pathways are essential for tumor cell growth. In one such recent study, Project Achilles, 102 human cell lines were screened for their dependence on 11,194 genes using short hairpin RNA knockdown.[18] Of these, 54 genes were found to be required for the proliferation of ovarian cancer cell lines that were either amplified or overexpressed in primary tumors. Similar

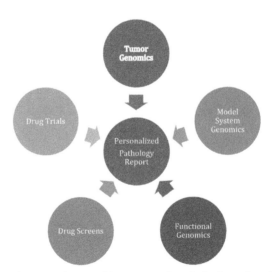

Fig. 5. Multipronged approach to making sense of pathologic and molecular data. Integrated pathology reports of the future will likely need to integrate disparate data sources to produce clinically meaningful and easily interpreted reports. Important aspects include identifying the driving genomic alterations in the tumor, comparison to genomic alterations present in various cell line models (*Model System Genomics*), prioritization of therapeutically significant mutations through integration with genome wide small interfering RNA studies (*Functional Genomics*) and drug screens performed in the correct genomic context, and identification of relevant clinical trials.

types of functional studies have been performed in breast cancer cell lines that have highlighted the importance of phosphoinositide 3-kinase signaling, which is of particular interest given the high frequency of *PIK3CA* mutations in breast cancer.[19] These kinds of data are likely to be incorporated into future reports to provide a rationale for highlighting mutations that are most likely to be therapeutically significant. An even more therapeutically relevant approach would be to incorporate the results of *Drug Screens* involving screening cell lines with clinically available drugs. In one such example, several hundred cell lines characterized by targeted sequencing and microarray expression analysis were tested for sensitivity to 130 drugs under preclinical or clinical investigation.[20] This study uncovered several frequently mutated genes that could be correlated with particular chemotherapy sensitivities, information that could be a valuable input for future reports. Future reports pointing toward specific therapies based on the molecular profile will ultimately require clinical validation and, short of that, some kind of assessment of the strength of the evidence for those conclusions. In addition, it is possible that pathologists will test cells from fresh tumor biopsy samples for sensitivity to a broad range of chemotherapies and reporting out their sensitivities to the drugs instead of having the clinicians perform these "experiments" in patients. These are not areas that pathologists have ventured into previously, so validation of these approaches will require considerable work and careful correlation of predictions with clinical follow-up. Another high value added aspect of pathology reports could be the analysis of *Drug Trials,* particularly the strength of the evidence that a particular type of tumor with a particular mutation will respond to a given chemotherapy. It would be convenient, for example, to have pathology reports that provide up-to-date information on what clinical trials are open and where they are located.

Regardless of the strategies used, improvements in reporting and patient care will depend on having a robust means of tracking both clinical outcomes of patients and given mutations in a sufficiently large group to have statistically valid results. Some early efforts include single-institution efforts such as that at the Dana Farber Cancer Center and privately led efforts such as that of the Genetic Care Interchange organized by Life Technologies. A large part of the success of any of these ventures will be to have therapies that will generate survival improvements that justify the considerable expense of going down this path.

MOVING TOWARD DIAGNOSTIC TEAMS

The days when one person has all of the knowledge and experience required to make complex interpretations may be over, at least in some areas. It is likely that team sign-out of reports is coming. As discussed earlier, the Michigan Oncology Sequencing Project initiative involves a diverse group of experts to analyze complex, genomewide sequencing results. It seems likely that teams of specialists will share sign-out responsibility in the future, which raises practical questions about who is reimbursed for what and by whom and who holds the primary medicolegal responsibility.

AN INCREASING ROLE FOR THE FOR-PROFIT SECTOR IN PATHOLOGY

A remarkable number of for-profit companies have begun offering pathology services, particularly in the area of molecular diagnostics. This raises important questions about the role of the on-site pathologist in future diagnostics. Competition for academic pathology laboratories comes not only from freestanding reference laboratories but increasingly from well-capitalized multinational corporations. In just a short period, GE's (Fairfield, CT) Healthcare division has purchased Clarient (Aliso Viejo, CA), a cancer diagnostics company; hired additional pathologists; and purchased SeqWright

(Houston, TX), a sequencing services company. Instrument makers such as Life Technologies (Carlsbad, CA) are working to commoditize sequencing-based diagnostics with products such as Ampliseq, a 46-oncogene panel sequenced on the Ion Torrent instrument. Several firms now offer multiplexed assays for guiding cancer therapy. Some of the more widely used tests attempt to predict which patients with early-stage breast cancer will benefit from systemic therapy and which are unlikely to benefit. These involve integrating multiple biomarkers into a single score to predict the likelihood of recurrence or metastasis. Two of the tests, MammaPrint by Agendia (Irvine, CA) and the Oncotype DX by Genomic Health (Redwood City, CA), combine measurements of messenger RNA from the tumor to define a risk score for recurrent breast cancer. Although these tests have some overlap in the biomarkers they incorporate, the MammaPrint test interrogates more targets and, in contrast to Oncotype DX, its use is not restricted to estrogen receptor or progesterone receptor–positive disease. In contrast to the MammaPrint and Oncotype DX tests, the MammaStrat test by Clarient uses 5 immunohistochemistry biomarkers weighted by an algorithm to determine low, medium, or high risk of recurrence. Like the Oncotype DX test, the MammaStrat test is restricted to estrogen receptor–positive breast cancers. One important difference between these tests is that the Oncotype DX not only produces a recurrence score but also has implications for the use of chemotherapy. A low score on the Oncotype DX indicates that the patient will not benefit from chemotherapy, whereas a high score is an indication that the patient will benefit from chemotherapy. Genomic Health has introduced an Oncotype DX–like test for colon cancer. By identifying which patients are more likely to benefit from chemotherapy, these tests have the potential to stratify the use of systemic therapy to improve the quality of life of patients with a low risk of recurrence by avoiding unnecessary chemotherapy. This approach has been explicitly shown to work for the Oncotype DX test but is more implicit in the information provided by the MammaPrint and MammaStrat. Other tests use RNA expression levels to determine the site of origin for a cancer with unknown primary location. Pathwork Diagnostics (Redwood City, CA) and bioTheranostics (San Diego, CA) both market tests based on messenger RNA content from formalin-fixed paraffin-embedded (FFPE) samples, whereas Rosetta Genomics (Rehovot, Israel) markets a test based on micro-RNA expression. Of note, the Pathwork test received Food and Drug Administration (FDA) approval in 2010. Several reference laboratories now offer biomarker panels for determining which drug(s) are likely to be effective on a particular tumor type (eg, a panel for lung cancer and a separate panel for colon cancer). With the proliferation of targeted therapies, performing such biomarker panels will become the standard of care and will be demanded by both patients and insurers of care. The Quest Diagnostics (Madison, NJ) lung cancer panel, for example, includes tests for *EGFR*, *ALK*, and *KRAS* mutation. Similarly, their colorectal cancer mutation panel includes tests for *NRAS, KRAS, PIK3CA,* and *BRAF*. Somewhat expanded panels for lung, colorectal, and gastric cancers are now available from Response Genetics (San Francisco, CA). More comprehensive tumor profiling services are also available that are generally targeted at late-stage patients for whom first-line therapy has failed and who seek guidance in selecting additional therapy that might be beneficial. Caris Life Sciences (Irving, TX) and Foundation Medicine (Cambridge, MA) offer tumor profiling services that combine panels of biomarkers culled from the literature. The test offered by Caris assesses the tumor's molecular pathways via protein detection, gene expression, fluorescence in situ hybridization, and limited mutational analysis, whereas the Foundation Medicine assays are based on next-generation sequencing of tumor DNA. These are reported back to the treating physician along with drug associations to assist the physician in making treatment decisions based on the unique biology of the tumor they are treating. These tests are limited in the number of biomarkers analyzed and they typically are used to interrogate the tumor at a single point in time, often at diagnosis instead of at relapse or metastasis. As was noted in a recent article in the *New England Journal of Medicine*,[21] the high mutational heterogeneity of many tumors poses major challenges in therapy selection, as resistance is likely to arise quickly from preexisting clones.

SERVICE STILL MATTERS – HOW DO WE BETTER SERVE THE END USER?

Pathology reports will continue to be primarily directed to clinicians. The more specific information about what the patient has, what the prognosis is, and what the most effective therapy is likely to be, the better will be the report. In the authors' experience in running a reference laboratory, the main drivers for customer satisfaction are turnaround time, having reports that are easy to navigate, and having a pathologist available to field calls whenever necessary. The typical clinician is busy and will be even more challenged in the future trying to process large amounts of information. A revealing article in the *New England Journal of Medicine* assessed the activities of physicians in a busy primary care practice.[22] The results were sobering. The typical physician's day included an average of 18.1 patient visits, 23.7 telephone calls, 12.1 prescription refills, 16.8 e-mails, 19.5 lab report reviews, 11.1 imaging report reviews, and 13.9 consultant report reviews.

Clearly, many clinicians are stretched to the limit. It is difficult to imagine how they will have time to make sense of 20 pathology reports per day that include large panels of molecular diagnostic results. Pathologists will do well to make the reports as informative and understandable as possible. Many helpful guidelines have been offered to improve the quality of reports.[23,24] Diagnostic headlines can be used in newspaper format to convey the most important information at the top in the largest font followed by subheadings conveying more specific information. Just as the 6 essential instruments in airplanes are organized in the same way, the different elements of reports can be organized in a way that is consistent from report to report over time. Current reports are often lacking in that they remain fragmented. Making a note to "see flow cytometry report" is just adding another to-do item to the busy clinician's work list. The surgical pathology report of the future will need to have all of the ancillary data and a discussion of the implications of the findings integrated into one report. One pathologist, generally the one who reviews the histology, would be responsible for integrating the data and issuing the final diagnosis. This could be implemented by having a preliminary diagnosis, and then when all of the additional data are available, the pathologist is prompted by the laboratory information system to issue a final interpretation of all the data. With the increasing complexity of data, particularly molecular genetic data, this integration will become more and more important.

Clinicians, of course, are not the only ones who read pathology reports. Patients are already increasingly requesting their reports and contacting pathologists with questions. The Health Information Technology for Economic and Clinical Health Act will only make this more commonplace as the act requires that patients have access to their medical records through a patient portal. Some institutions have developed user-friendly Web sites to provide information useful to both patients and clinicians. Vanderbilt University's My Cancer Genome Web site (www.mycancergenome.org), for example, provides a portal for looking up common cancer types and the mutations associated with them. The links provide additional information on the frequency of specific mutations and their predicted responsiveness to different types of chemotherapy along with associated references. The site also provides links to clinical trials that are registered with PDQ and clinicaltrials.gov. These will be standard features of first-rate pathology reports in the future.

AN INCREASING ROLE FOR FEDERAL REGULATION

As more multiplexed tests have been introduced, the FDA has shown increasing interest in their regulation. The FDA recently issued draft guidelines on, for example, in vitro diagnostic multivariate index assays (IVDMIAs), which are defined as devices "that: (1) combines the values of multiple variables using an interpretation function to yield a single, patient-specific result (eg, a "classification," "score," "index," etc.), that is intended for the diagnosis of disease or other conditions, or in the cure, mitigation, treatment or prevention of disease, and (2) provides a result whose derivation is non-transparent and cannot be independently derived or verified by the end user." (www.fda.gov/MedicalDevices/DeviceRegulationandGuidance/GuidanceDocuments/UCM 079148.htm). Furthermore, the agency stipulates that they reserve the right to review these assays. To date, the FDA has not required all IVDMIA tests be submitted for review (the Agendia and Pathwork tests were voluntarily submitted and approved) but it remains to be seen how big a role the agency will play in policing the IVDMIA marketplace in the future. If this role is aggressive, it may become increasingly difficult for academic laboratories to offer the multiplexed assays because of the lack of resources required to secure full FDA approval. Pathology sign-out in the future may also be heavily affected by gene patenting, a topic that cannot be done justice in this brief review. In short, the more intellectual property holders try to operate as the exclusive service providers or sign exclusive patent licensing deals, the more difficult it will be for reference laboratories to offer the full range of services necessary. During the next decade, it seems likely that there will be legislation curtailing exclusive testing rights and perhaps more gene patent pools to prevent gene patents from becoming a major obstacle to better patient care.

HOW CAN PATHOLOGY BEND THE COST CURVE?

Although the increasingly sophisticated diagnostic testing repertoire is promising, it is clear that current health care spending levels are unsustainable. It would not be surprising if pathology services are one of the first places payers turn to for cuts, so pathologists will do well to articulate the value proposition that their testing provides. Some areas of particular opportunity could include prostate cancer, where better biomarkers and risk prevention models might reduce the frequency of biopsies and, when tumors are discovered, provide more accurate decision support on whether a prostatectomy is warranted. It also seems likely that much of anatomic pathology will become digitized. This creates new opportunities for outreach (as well as potential revenue loss through outsourcing of pathology services) and the possibility of deploying expertise between institutions when volumes do not warrant hiring a full-time subspecialty pathologist.

TIME FOR NEW BUSINESS MODELS

Academic and community pathology departments, as currently configured, are not well poised to meet the future demands of diagnostic pathology, particularly in the area of molecular pathology and high-throughput sequencing. If the departments do not operate an outreach laboratory, it is unlikely that they will have the volumes required to make "insourcing" tests cost effective. Under intense cost constraints, clinical pathology laboratories are staffed at levels just sufficient to meet day-to-day needs, with little "bandwidth" in most departments for the sophisticated research and development required for new assay development. Capital budgeting processes are slow and involve innumerable tradeoffs with other units with pressing concerns. Faculty in academic medical centers find themselves struggling to fulfill their disparate missions, yet in the outreach arena, they are competing with well-capitalized competitors staffed by full-time employees dedicated to clinical care. And, at the macro level, the idea that each medical center will operate a high-end molecular diagnostics laboratory, with the level of information technology infrastructure required, seems increasingly implausible.

All of these factors point to the likelihood that high-end pathologic testing will become increasingly consolidated, the main question being whether testing will continue to be done in the academic sector or if much of this work will be done in large reference laboratories and specialized for-profit corporations such as those described earlier. One model that shows promise is the cotenancy laboratory, in which several medical centers pool resources and operate one reference laboratory staffed by full-time pathologists and technologists, such as Warde Medical Laboratories in Ann Arbor, Michigan, the largest cotenancy laboratory in the United States. Spreading fixed costs over a higher volume and taking advantage of economies of scale on supplies make it possible to reduce overall operating costs and offer a wider range of services. In addition, the model is financially attractive. Instead of laboratories facing ever rising send-out costs, it preserves the rights of "cotenants" to bill for services provided on a cost-plus basis. Still another alternative for providing services are academic–industry hybrid laboratories, in which the pathology department partners with another academic medical center or corporate partner to provide the particular expertise or infrastructure that is lacking.

Closing Thoughts

Technologies and business models change quickly. Nothing is a given—what pathologists do today is likely to be very different in the future. The advent of high-end molecular testing is a great opportunity if pathologists respond proactively to the themes outlined in this report. However, if they do not, they may find themselves in a much less desirable world 20 years from now, disintermediated and no longer playing the central role they once did in guiding patient care.

REFERENCES

1. Grasso CS, Wu YM, Robinson DR, et al. The mutational landscape of lethal castrate resistant prostate cancer. Nature 2012;487(7406):239–43.
2. Taylor BS, Schultz N, Hieronymus H, et al. Integrative genomic profiling of human prostate cancer. Cancer Cell 2010;18(1):11–22.
3. Tomlins SA, Mehra R, Rhodes DR, et al. Integrative molecular concept modeling of prostate cancer progression. Nat Genet 2007;39(1):41–51.
4. Maher CA, Kumar-Sinha C, Cao X, et al. Transcriptome sequencing to detect gene fusions in cancer. Nature 2009;458(7234):97–101.
5. Maher CA, Palanisamy N, Brenner JC, et al. Chimeric transcript discovery by paired-end transcriptome sequencing. Proc Natl Acad Sci U S A 2009;106(30):12353–8.
6. Prensner JR, Iyer MK, Balbin OA, et al. Transcriptome sequencing across a prostate cancer cohort identifies PCAT-1, an unannotated lincRNA implicated in disease progression. Nat Biotechnol 2011;29(8):742–9.

7. Berger MF, Lawrence MS, Demichelis F, et al. The genomic complexity of primary human prostate cancer. Nature 2011;470(7333):214–20.

8. Fong PC, Boss DS, Yap TA, et al. Inhibition of poly(ADP-ribose) polymerase in tumors from BRCA mutation carriers. N Engl J Med 2009;361(2):123–34.

9. Roberts PJ, Bisi JE, Strum JC, et al. Multiple roles of cyclin-dependent kinase 4/6 inhibitors in cancer therapy. J Natl Cancer Inst 2012;104(6):476–87.

10. Attard G, Reid AH, Olmos D, et al. Antitumor activity with CYP17 blockade indicates that castration-resistant prostate cancer frequently remains hormone driven. Cancer Res 2009;69(12):4937–40.

11. Shen MM, Abate-Shen C. Molecular genetics of prostate cancer: new prospects for old challenges. Genes Dev 2010;24(18):1967–2000.

12. Attard G, de Bono JS. Utilizing circulating tumor cells: challenges and pitfalls. Curr Opin Genet Dev 2011;21(1):50–8.

13. Sarker D, Reid AH, Yap TA, et al. Targeting the PI3K/AKT pathway for the treatment of prostate cancer. Clin Cancer Res 2009;15(15):4799–805.

14. Cakir M, Grossman AB. Medullary thyroid cancer: molecular biology and novel molecular therapies. Neuroendocrinology 2009;90(4):323–48.

15. Pao W, Hutchinson KE. Chipping away at the lung cancer genome. Nat Med 2012;18(3):349–51.

16. Wells SA Jr, Robinson BG, Gagel RF, et al. Vandetanib in patients with locally advanced or metastatic medullary thyroid cancer: a randomized, double-blind phase III trial. J Clin Oncol 2012;30(2):134–41.

17. Roychowdhury S, Iyer MK, Robinson DR, et al. Personalized oncology through integrative high-throughput sequencing: a pilot study. Sci Transl Med 2011; 3(111):111–21.

18. Cheung HW, Cowley GS, Weir BA, et al. Systematic investigation of genetic vulnerabilities across cancer cell lines reveals lineage-specific dependencies in ovarian cancer. Proc Natl Acad Sci U S A 2011;108(30):12372–7.

19. Brough R, Frankum JR, Sims D, et al. Functional viability profiles of breast cancer. Cancer Discov 2011;1(3):260–73.

20. Garnett MJ, Edelman EJ, Heidorn SJ, et al. Systematic identification of genomic markers of drug sensitivity in cancer cells. Nature 2012;483(7391):570–5.

21. Gerlinger M, Rowan AJ, Horswell S, et al. Intratumor heterogeneity and branched evolution revealed by multiregion sequencing. N Engl J Med 2012;366(10): 883–92.

22. Baron RJ. What's keeping us so busy in primary care? A snapshot from one practice. N Engl J Med 2010;362(17):1632–6.

23. Valenstein PN. Formatting pathology reports: applying four design principles to improve communication and patient safety. Arch Pathol Lab Med 2008;132(1): 84–94.

24. Hess JL. What hematopathology tells us about the future of pathology informatics. Arch Pathol Lab Med 2009;133(6):908–11.

Changing Trends in Laboratory Testing in the United States

A Personal, Historical Perspective

Charles M. Strom, MD, PhD, HCLD, CQ (NY), Cert Dir (CA), diplomate ABMG(CG, CBCG, CMG)

KEYWORDS

- Academic laboratory • Commercial laboratory • Business of pathology

KEY POINTS

- Changes in the economic and academic landscape parallel technological innovations in laboratory testing.
- Clinical laboratory testing is a multibillion dollar industry that, in the United States, is dominated by two giant national clinical laboratories.
- Although the academic laboratory is under heavy pressure, innovative joint ventures with commercial entities, both in clinical testing and in education can potentially ensure their survival.

INTRODUCTION

This article contains a series of mostly personal "Aha!" moments that are exclamation points along the time line of changing trends in laboratory testing in the United States. I hope readers find this account entertaining and informative, elucidating the scientific and economic selection processes that impact the system in the evolution of genetic testing.

The opinions expressed in this article are my own and do not reflect the positions of any company, association, or entity. This is not a research paper. If I have used an incorrect date or made a misstatement, I apologize and will stand corrected. This is a synthesis of events as I experienced them.

To engage in meaningful, informed discussion, it is vital to have a clear definition of terms. The following definitions explain some of the terms I use in this article as my frame of reference:

> Commercial laboratory—a commercial entity founded to make a profit performing laboratory tests. These laboratories usually have a sales and/or marketing staff

Genetics, Quest Diagnostics Nichols Institute, 33608 Ortega Highway, San Juan Capistrano, CA 92675-2042, USA
E-mail address: Charles.M.Strom@QuestDiagnostics.com

Clin Lab Med 32 (2012) 651–664
http://dx.doi.org/10.1016/j.cll.2012.07.003
0272-2712/12/$ – see front matter © 2012 Elsevier Inc. All rights reserved.

who are trained to sell laboratory testing to providers and health plans. Commercial laboratories solicit testing on a national and, sometimes, international scope.

Academic laboratory—a university hospital–based, primary research, grant-supported laboratory that may or may not perform diagnostic testing for patients.

Hybrid laboratory—a commercial laboratory affiliated with an academic medical center or institution of higher education.

Regional laboratory—for-profit laboratories that are usually affiliated with a regional hospital network to centralize laboratory services for cost-saving purposes. These laboratories often provide services for health plan patients and for outreach clinics of their affiliated institutions, and compete with national commercial and hybrid laboratories in their catchment areas.

Focused commercial laboratory—a national commercial laboratory that concentrates on a single disease state or medical specialty, sometimes performing a single test based on intellectual property exclusivity. Often these companies are spin-offs from academic centers created to commercialize a particular test or technology.

Community hospital laboratory—a laboratory that predominantly provides service to patients from its own medical facilities (ie, "mom and pop" laboratories)

Academic medical center—hospitals and clinics affiliated with a medical school or other institute of higher education.

House officers, house staff—interns, residents, and postdoctoral fellows practicing within an academic hospital setting.

Esoteric test—there really is no universally accepted definition of an esoteric test. For the purposes of this article, I define it as a test that is technically beyond the capabilities of most hospital-based laboratories. I have heard an esoteric test defined as a test with a greater than 20% profit margin, but I prefer the former definition.

Laboratory developed test—a test independently designed and validated by a laboratory that is specific to that laboratory.

Translational medicine—a new field of endeavor encouraging transitions from basic research to clinical utility.

A HISTORY OF GENETIC TESTING: A MODEL OF NATURAL SELECTION?

Darwinian theory requires two forces to be at work, the potential for change and pressures causing natural selection. There is no doubt about the ability of individuals, organizations, and systems to adapt, so this article focuses on the selective forces that pressured genetics laboratories to adapt.

2012

Clinical laboratory testing is a multibillion dollar industry dominated by two giant national clinical laboratories, Quest Diagnostics and the Laboratory Corporation of America. These laboratories perform high-throughput testing in all genetic specialties. Hybrid laboratories affiliated with academic centers have become national commercial entities. Hybrid and commercial laboratories currently perform most high-volume genetic testing. The small, single-disease, academic laboratory, is nearly extinct. Focused commercial laboratories are replacing their function in performing cutting edge testing.[1]

The Center for Medicare/Medicaid Services, Clinical Laboratory Improvement Act (CLIA), the College of American Pathologists, the Food and Drug Administration (FDA), and various state Departments of Health are all involved in one way or another in the oversight and regulation of the laboratory testing industry (see the long list of credentials required for me to be a Laboratory Director next to my name).[1] Tests move from publication to bedside so quickly that a new branch of medical science called translational medicine has been created. How did we get here? I propose: by a process of selection and adaptation, with a combination of forces acting on the system to cause its inevitable evolution.

THE PRIMORDIAL OOZE, OR PRE-1968

In the beginning, there were no large centralized commercial testing laboratories or laboratory regulation. Nearly all routine laboratory tests were performed by community hospital pathologists in what my generation affectionately calls "mom and pop" laboratories. Most esoteric testing was performed in academic medical centers either in their centralized laboratories or in individual grant-supported research laboratories specializing in a particular disease or family of diseases.

Before the molecular era (pre-1975), most genetic testing consisted of analyte assays or enzyme assays. Amino acid quantitation (developed in the late 1950s) using amino acid analyzers, and organic acid analysis (developed in the early 1960s) using gas chromatograpy and/or mass spectrometry, and glycosaminoglycan analysis by thin layer chromatography (developed in the early 1960s) were the archetypical analyte tests. The hemoglobinopathies were diagnosed using hemoglobin electrophoresis (developed in the 1960s) and alpha-1-antitrypsin deficiency by two-dimensional gel electrophoresis. These tests were all performed in academic medical centers in specialized laboratories within the institutions. If the analyte tests suggested a specific diagnosis, individual laboratories performed confirmatory enzyme analysis. Often just one laboratory in the world performed this specialized assay.

As cytogenetics emerged, specialized laboratories performed prenatal (1970s) and postnatal (1960s) karyotyping. Molecular diagnostics was in its infancy. In 1982, Y.W. Kan described prenatal diagnosis for sickle cell anemia.[2]

There was no centralized genetics laboratory in the institution where I worked in the early 1980s. Organic acids were run in the neurology department, amino acids in pediatrics, karyotypes in obstetrics-gynecology (OB-GYN), and enzyme analysis was scattered throughout the Joseph P. Kennedy Mental Retardation Center located on the upper floors of the Wyler Children's Hospital.

Part of the art of practicing Clinical Genetics was knowing which academic laboratory throughout the world performed the requisite testing for each patient. Because there was no external regulation yet, any graduate student with a pipette and fluorimeter could deliver clinical test results. Because academic laboratories were primarily funded by their research grants, genetic testing was performed to advance research and to optimize patient care instead of as a profit-making enterprise.

1974: Aha Moment Number One

As a young, Jewish, married, graduate student, I was eager to be tested for Tay-Sachs disease carrier status. The laboratory performing the test was part of the same program project grant as my mentor was. I asked the laboratory director how I could get tested. He directed me to a laboratory tech who taught me the assay. Then I drew my own blood and tested it myself. Today, such a practice would violate several statutes and regulations (the Health Insurance Portability and Accountability Act [HIPPAA] and CLIA, to name a couple).

My realization: in 1974, anybody could do laboratory testing!

And the Testing World Was Without Form

Temperatures of water baths and incubators were rarely, if ever, checked. Centrifuges went uncalibrated and we mouth-pipetted reagents and patient samples using glass or sometimes disposable plastic pipettes. Reports were often handwritten and, sometimes, illegible and/or undecipherable. Laboratory recordkeeping was haphazard, with patient results often buried in laboratory notebooks covered with water spots and undecipherable comments. A standard operating procedure was an alien concept.

Because generating income was not the primary motivation of university laboratories, billing and payment for services was sporadic and erratic. Patients or the ordering physician might receive enormous invoices several months after testing was performed. Most unpaid bills went uncollected because academic laboratories did not have formal billing departments. Some laboratories, such as ours, initially charged no fees at all for testing.

1978: Aha Moment Number Two

My wife and I were trying to conceive our first child. I had just attended a medical student lecture describing a newly developed radioimmunoassay (RIA) for human chorionic gonadotropin. The following morning, I drew my wife's blood at home and hand carried it to the endocrine research laboratory where they happily accepted it with no paperwork. When I returned the following day, I received smiles and congratulations from my colleagues (another HIPAA violation, of course). No bill, no paperwork, just hugs!

Realization: new research and development developments can rapidly be introduced into the clinical environment for the benefit of the patient.

LET THERE BE PROFITS

For me, the scientific environment changed when academic medical centers began to choose individuals with a business background to run hospitals and clinical services — instead of academicians and physicians.

Historically, there was little pressure on academic medical centers to be profitable, or even to break even. They were considered prestigious assets, vital to the success of a university's mandate to educate medical students and house officers. Financial shortfalls were often subsidized by the parent institution. Academic medical centers were run by academic scientists and physicians whose main concerns were research, the quality of patient care, and teaching in their facilities.

The salaries of most of the attending physicians were paid by salary support from research grants and the institution received compensation for supporting its laboratory facilities by collecting indirect costs from the granting bodies. There was no distinction between clinical and academic faculty. As an assistant professor of pediatrics, I wrote grants, taught undergraduates and medical students, and mentored graduate students and postdoctoral fellows. I also attended on the wards 2 months each year. The Genetics Clinic met once a week in the Pediatric Department and I participated in the prenatal diagnosis program in the OB-GYN department.

Academic laboratories had multiple functions and clinical testing was the least important. The primary goal of a laboratory in the early 1980s was to perform scientific research. Ideally, this would result in peer-reviewed publications written by the scientists, grant renewal, and, perhaps, tenure for the laboratory director and/or principal investigator. A secondary function was educating medical students and house officers. Clinical service to patients was a related, but unequal, priority.

Increasing economic pressure on universities created the necessity for more fiscal discipline in general. Universities began to look at their attached medical centers and clinics as a potential source of revenue and not just an extension of their educational campuses.

Changes in the economic and regulatory climate, and the explosion of technological innovations in human genetics, exerted pressure to adapt. This led to a transformation in genetic testing. The time trends for these forces overlap; the order in which they are presented is somewhat arbitrary, based on my experience. These selection forces fall into three categories: economic, regulatory, and technological. Economic forces include academic medical centers evolving into profit centers, health care cost containment, reduction in grant support, intellectual property, and changes in reimbursement for testing.[3]

SELECTION FORCE NUMBER ONE: ECONOMIC PRESSURE
The Academic Medical Center as Profit Center

1984: Aha moment number three
Our hospital hired a "business type" as the new executive director. He convened a meeting to discuss billing issues. The discussion turned to maternity services. After several questions, it was determined that nobody knew if we were billing for any of the circumcisions performed on newborn boys in our hospital. It turned out, we were not. This was followed-up by a discussion of whether the foreskin could (not should) be sent to Pathology for review and, hence, generate another potential lucrative fee. It was eventually a split decision: yes to billing for circumcision, no to sending the foreskin to pathology.

Realization: we were not in the Ivory Tower (Kansas) anymore. Publications and grant support were replaced by revenue as the currency de jour.

The hospital laboratory became a cash cow with potential to generate large profits for the university. Although the Pathology Department had a centralized laboratory to perform routine testing and anatomic pathology services, esoteric testing was, for the most part, spread throughout the campus in specialized grant-supported academic laboratories.

Given the mandate to generate higher revenues, university hospitals and clinics expanded their roles beyond research and teaching. Administrators were not content with a minimum number of patient visits and admissions needed to fulfill an educational mission. To increase profits, the number of patient visits and admissions had to increase. A staff of full-time, research-oriented physician-scientists, supported by grants, who attended in the wards and clinics a few months a year, was inadequate. Almost every major academic medical center began to hire clinical faculty to satisfy the increased patient loads. Instead of being judged on the success of their scientific research (winning grants and publishing results), faculty would be judged on revenue generation and teaching.

As the number of clinic visits and hospitalizations increased exponentially in the 1990s, it became imperative to operate centralized clinical laboratories staffed by full-time professionals (usually pathologists). Automated analyzers were developed to allow high-quality, high-throughput testing with minimal staffing requirements. For the most part, however, genetic services continued to be scattered throughout academic campuses.

A particularly thorny issue was what to do about genetic testing. As noted above, several different physical laboratories in several different departments provided genetic testing services. The Pathology Department argued vociferously that these laboratories should be centralized into their core laboratory structure. This notion was summarily dismissed by the cytogeneticists and biochemical geneticists, who argued that their unique expertise was crucial to appropriate testing and interpretation of cytogenetic results.

Thus began the ongoing 50-year cytogenetics war between pathologists and geneticists about control of cytogenetics laboratories. Although there are intermittent cease-fires and peace treaties, hostilities were always just beneath the surface, ready to heat up with any change in administration or personnel. In every institution I have worked in or visited, the genetics–pathology tug-of-war over cytogenetics continues.

Regardless of who achieved the upper hand, the days when an individual laboratory could report out a result without billing for it were over. Even though the laboratories might remain physically scattered throughout the academic campus, centralized billing and collection departments were created. Whether the individual laboratories received any benefit from their generated revenue was dependant on the organizational structure.

1994: Aha moment number four

I attended a cocktail reception at a professional conference and entered into a discussion with a clinical pathologist who ran a hospital laboratory. He proudly confided in me that it cost him less than $5.00 to run a "Chem 20" panel and he was billing $60.00 and receiving full reimbursement.

Realization: thar is gold in them-there laboratory tests!

Health Care Cost Containment: Expulsion from the Garden

The days when genetic testing was a research tool to advance scientific knowledge, when tests were paid for by grant-supported research and were free from outside scrutiny, were coming to an end.

Almost unnoticed by the academic world, a new entity was born: the large commercial testing laboratory. In 1968, MetPath (New York City, London, England) was founded to provide laboratory testing services to a national clientele. The following year, the pharmaceutical company SmithKline Beecham acquired eight testing laboratories and combined them into a single administrative entity (eventually, both Met Path and SmithKline were acquired by Quest Diagnostics). By 1975, MetPath was one of the largest testing laboratories in the world. Most routine laboratory testing was performed using automated analyzers that allowed higher throughput, consistent results, and lower costs than manual testing.

In other developments, academicians began to leave universities to open for-profit testing laboratories using the latest technologies such as radioimmunoassays. Almost as fast as these laboratories became profitable, a commercial laboratory purchased them. Commercial laboratories could acquire esoteric testing capabilities in this way.

In 1982, MetPath installed computer terminals in physician offices that were connected to its laboratory's main computer system, allowing physicians to receive results instantaneously. This ushered in the era of information on demand that we have become so accustomed to in the twenty-first century.

The founding of Alfigen in 1980 and Genzyme in 1981 changed the genetic testing landscape. These national commercial laboratories were founded to provide esoteric genetic testing services to a national clientele. The gauntlet was thrown down: could universities remain at the forefront of genetic testing? Academic laboratories were slow to notice that a change in priorities from research, teaching, and patient care to profits would naturally select for commercial laboratories. Why would anyone prefer to send samples to a commercial entity, some anonymous, nonacademic "stranger," instead of to state-of-the-art academic laboratories?

As of 1999, a review concluded, "In conclusion, our study demonstrates that genetic testing facilities in the US are still a heterogeneous group. The field as a whole seems to be far from dominated by any of the involved players. According to our data, academic laboratories were the most common institution type and performed the largest share (64%) of molecular-genetic tests. These results also show that molecular-genetic testing is still largely a cottage industry in the US, with test volumes that are minuscule compared with most other parts of the clinical laboratory."[4]

Academic scientists were certain that a centralized laboratory could not possibly provide the same high-quality services as their own laboratories. Surely, these start-ups would soon fade away. The sale of Genzyme Genetics to the Laboratory Corporation of America for more than $700 million 30 years later proves just how flawed our thinking turned out to be.

In the early 1980s, as commercial laboratories were beginning to get a foothold, academia did not really take the competition seriously. Why? There was still enough money to go around. Medical costs continued to rise unchecked and no one really bothered to make cheaper testing a priority because the costs could be passed along to patients in terms of higher insurance premiums or the government in terms of Medicaid and Medicare billing. Academic centers had an advantage because their Medicare and Medicaid reimbursement rates were higher than in nonteaching hospitals as a compensation for their role in educating medical students and house officers.

A few academic laboratories spun off their own commercial laboratory entities, ushering in the concept of a hybrid laboratory, but, by and large, the academic genetics laboratories continued to ignore competition from the commercial laboratories despite a progressive erosion of their testing volume.

In addition to the competition from commercial laboratories, other corollary forces began to pressure the academic genetic testing laboratory: reduced grant support, health care cost containment, regulatory intervention, and financial competition.

Reduction in Grant Support

An inevitable decline occurred in grant funding for primary research laboratories performing clinical genetic testing. Initially, the principal investigator would secure grant funding to explore a particular disease or family of diseases. This would be followed by the delineation of the mechanism of the disease, often leading to a clinical diagnostic test. After several years, the problem was considered solved and funding became more difficult to obtain and was eventually lost. The laboratory relied on income from testing or support from the parent institution to remain solvent. Even when grants were funded, the research plan did not include clinical testing. So, if the laboratory director decided to continue to perform clinical testing, resources would have to be diverted from the basic research. The overall increased competition for grant support and reduced funding sources exacerbated these challenges.

Intellectual Property: It's My Ball and You Can't Play

In the early 1980s, the Reagan Administration decided to encourage universities and other receivers of federal government sponsored research to aggressively pursue patents for inventions created with taxpayer money. The patent office was encouraged to allow patents for biologic processes. They reasoned that this privatization of research could wean universities from their reliance on federal funds and encourage a private sector to develop around these issued patents. This has created a climate in which almost every clinically relevant gene, mutation, or testing platform is patented. This has increased the cost of performing genetic testing because laboratories must obtain a license and pay royalties for almost every test performed. These fees are a significant cost of testing and make it difficult for smaller laboratories to offer a complete menu of innovative tests.[5]

Health Care Cost Containment

In the "early days" there was little or no scrutiny of the costs of clinical laboratory testing. With the emergence of managed care and governmental scrutiny of Medicare and Medicaid fee-for-service costs, those days came to a screeching halt. Quickly, routine testing became a commodity. Major insurers negotiated prices with large commercial and regional laboratories. If the local hospital laboratory charged more for a test than a large commercial laboratory, then the managed care, preferred provider organization, or private insurer began to require that testing for insured patients must go through the cheaper commercial laboratory.

1996: Aha moment number five

As a hospital geneticist, I saw patients in an OB-GYN clinic in Chicago. There was a large erasable board covered with the names of various insurance companies and what tests they would cover. It was the insurance company, rather than the physician, that decided whether a patient should have a thin prep or regular placental alkaline phosphatase (PAP) smear, or could have an ultrasound examination.

Realization: medical decisions are no longer completely under my (the physician's) control!

A particularly restrictive arrangement with physicians and hospitals was capitation, in which a fixed amount of money was paid to a physician or hospital and, in return, the physician or hospital was financially responsible for the medical care of a specified number of individuals. Physicians and hospitals participating in capitated programs had an even greater incentive to limit the cost of laboratory testing. This was another driver for hospitals and physicians to get the lowest possible price for laboratory testing, and to limit the amount of testing if possible.

Another selection force in the early 1980s was the change in Medicare and Medicaid reimbursement from fee-for-service to Diagnosis-Related Groups. A hospital or physician received a fixed sum for the diagnosis code or codes entered for the patient, not on the use of resources or the actual cost of providing care. Hospitals realized that expensive testing could result in a net loss for any given patient. Also in the early 1980s, the reimbursement of teaching hospitals became dissociated from the Medicare and Medicaid billing process. The result was an enormous financial incentive to minimize laboratory testing costs because they were not reimbursed.[6]

When I admitted a Medicare-insured patient with a bleeding ulcer, the hospital received the same reimbursement whether I monitored his or her blood counts hourly or daily. A system of financial credentialing was instituted in some hospitals, in which admitting physicians were monitored. If their patients' admissions resulted in a net loss to the hospital, the physician was given a warning. If this continued, admitting privileges could be revoked.

1998: Aha moment number six

At a medical staff meeting, our hospital comptroller announced that we were, on average, losing more than $200 each day for Medicare patients and, therefore, next year's goal was to limit Medicare admissions to 20% of patient days.

Realization: under certain circumstances, it is cheaper to not care for a patient than to care for a patient, or how screwed up is this?

Reimbursement

Molecular testing, although still considered esoteric, was evolving into a commodity. Until then, reimbursement for molecular testing was based on stacking of Current Procedural Technology (CPT) codes. CPT codes describe the technical procedures used for a specific assay. Each code has a corresponding expected reimbursement price. Therefore, a molecular assay might stack the following codes: DNA purification, polymerase chain reaction (PCR) amplification, restriction enzyme digestion, and capillary size separation. The industry has become accustomed to reimbursement based on these CPT codes. However, beginning in 2013, reimbursement for molecular testing will move from procedure-based stacked CPT coding to analyte-specific CPT coding. Reimbursement will be based on the mutation being analyzed instead of on the procedures used to generate the result. Although the reimbursement rates have not yet been established, no one expects them to increase with this system, placing even more pressure on smaller laboratories for cost containment.

SELECTION FORCE NUMBER TWO: REGULATORY REQUIREMENTS, OR THE COMMANDMENTS

In 1992, the clinical testing world was forever changed by the enactment of the CLIA. Before CLIA, any graduate student, postdoctoral fellow, or laboratory technician could perform a genetic test, report the results and bill for those services. CLIA defined three levels of laboratory testing: low, moderate, and high complexity. Low-complexity and moderate-complexity testing could usually be performed in a physician's office using FDA-cleared test kits.

High-complexity laboratory testing includes almost all genetic testing. The regulations specified requirements for the degrees and qualifications for laboratory directors and testing personnel, quality assurance, continuous quality improvement, record-keeping and many other facets of laboratory testing. CLIA mandates biannual inspections, proficiency testing, and many tasks unfamiliar to the small academic laboratories. Many academic laboratories had a difficult time adapting to the CLIA regulations. Daily monitoring of temperatures in water baths, periodic calibrating of pipettes and centrifuges, licensing of personnel, labeling of reagents with open dates and expiration dates, and massive documentation of training and competency made compliance with CLIA requirements an expensive and daunting task.

New York and California began regulating genetic testing separately from CLIA, causing even more cost and paperwork. Many academic laboratories simply decided to stop performing clinical testing. Others realized that to meet these standards, they would have to increase their test menus and test volumes to defray the cost of complying with CLIA regulations. Thus, hybrid laboratories such as Mayo Clinical Laboratories (Rochester, MN), Associated Regional and University Pathologists (Salt Lake City, Utah), and Boston College Genetics Laboratories (Boston, MA) began to hire sales and marketing staff, and increase menus and operational efficiencies to compete with the large commercial laboratories. These hybrid laboratories have a lot more in common with commercial laboratories than their ancestor, the academic laboratory.

SELECTION FORCE NUMBER THREE: TECHNOLOGICAL INNOVATION

When molecular testing was in its infancy, there was a single technique, the Southern blot (developed in 1975). Southern blots took weeks to perform, required radioactivity (P^{32}), and often needed to be repeated before getting interpretable results. Other hybridization technologies using allele-specific oligonucleotides were introduced to simplify matters somewhat. However, dot blots, slot blots, and reverse dot blots were still tedious, time consuming, and difficult to interpret. Central pathology laboratories were content to allow individual genetic research laboratories to perform this testing.

Before the description of PCR in 1983, molecular diagnostics required enormous technical skill, used radioactive labeling, and required significant expertise for review and interpretation. As recently as 1990, even after 7 years of PCR, almost all molecular diagnostics was based on gel electrophoresis or filter paper hybridization. These techniques were not easily adaptable to automation or large scale batching.

2000: Aha Moment Number Seven

I had just begun my new job as the medical director for molecular testing at a commercial laboratory. A scientist asked me if I would like to review the data of a platform comparison between our current dot blot technique and a new method based on mass spectrometry. I enthusiastically agreed. One thousand individuals had been analyzed for two different variants using both platforms. In the 1000 people and 2000 genotype calls, there had been 10 discrepancies. DNA-sequencing analysis had been performed on the 10 discrepant samples to determine the correct genotype. The bottom line was that our current dot blot assay was incorrect three times and the mass spectroscopy assay was incorrect seven times in these thousand samples. The scientist was pleased, believing we had vindicated our current method. I, however, was horrified because we were performing tens of thousands of tests each year and the review suggested we were giving people incorrect results a few dozen times per year.

This made me realize that:

1. Molecular techniques suitable for low-volume testing are not necessarily suitable for a high-throughput laboratory. Both platforms had error rates below 1% (0.15% and 0.35% for dot blot and mass spectroscopy, respectively) but, in high-throughput testing, this is not nearly good enough.
2. New platforms must be tested with at least 1000 samples to assess their technical accuracy because the standard 100-test benchmark is insufficient to assure the platform is accurate enough for high-throughput testing.[7,8]
3. It is imperative to discover methods that make no errors in 1000 samples to be confident of accuracy.

In the past two decades, a plethora of high-throughput, automated, easily interpretable platforms have become available. FDA-cleared test kits are available for the most common molecular tests such as cystic fibrosis carrier testing and thrombophilia testing. The advent of the automated capillary sequencer has allowed Sanger DNA sequencing to become a commonly ordered laboratory test.[9]

THE CURRENT STATUS: COMMERCIAL CONTRASTED WITH ACADEMIC LABORATORIES

The key to the success of commercial laboratories is volume, volume, volume. Of course, to generate and keep high volumes, testing accuracy and service levels must remain satisfactory. Generating large testing volumes allows several mechanisms to come into play:

1. Buying power. Because assays are performed at high volumes, commercial laboratories are able to negotiate favorable pricing with vendors, thereby significantly reducing costs per test.
2. Automation. Many tests can be performed simultaneously, usually in 96-well or 386-well microtiter plates. Automated DNA preparation instruments for isolating DNA, and automated liquid handlers, can be used for all pipetting steps, allowing a single laboratory technologist to generate results for a large number of patients by setting up and loading instruments instead of performing the manual tasks of pipetting. Because humans are prone to making errors while performing repetitive tasks, automation also decreases the likelihood of errors of sample switching or reagent addition (also see quality assurance).
3. Information technology (IT). Analytic platforms designed for plate-based assays can be chosen and interfaced with laboratory information systems to eliminate transcription errors. Because the data is transferred to the director's desktop

and a provisional genotype assignment made, the directors need only to review the quality data and correct any miscalls. When reading the results of proficiency testing, most of the errors are due to transcriptional errors, meaning the correct result was obtained but somebody filled in the form incorrectly. IT solutions can eliminate this as a source of error for clinical results.

4. Quality assurance. Large volume allows the laboratory to perform statistical analysis to detect any drift in the assay. If several thousand tests are performed each month, the percentage of genotype results should remain within a relatively tight window. By monitoring these genotypes, one can assure that the assay is performing as designed.

Commercial laboratories can perform high-volume genetic testing more cheaply and with higher quality than a low-volume laboratory. They have other significant advantages over academic laboratories:

1. Relationships with insurers. Because commercial laboratories offer an enormous menu of both routine and esoteric tests, they can offer one-stop-shopping to large insurers.
2. Service centers. Because of their size, commercial laboratories can offer service centers for patients to have their laboratory work performed.
3. Logistics. Commercial laboratories have fleets of vehicles (sometime including aircraft) to pick up specimens from hospitals and physician offices with the ability to transport those samples to a centralized location for testing.
4. Interfacing. Commercial laboratories are able to communicate directly to hospitals and physician's offices through direct links or web-based methods.
5. Sales force. Commercial laboratories have sales people who visit health care providers and hospitals, offering support, information, and access to their company's tests.
6. Marketing. Commercial laboratories have marketing departments who inform health care providers of their tests and tout the advantages of their company's tests over the competition.
7. Billing. Timely billing and collections are absolutely necessary to get reimbursement in the current competitive economic environment. It helps to have an efficient, organized system for billing and reimbursement.

1986: Aha Moment Number Eight—Blast from the Past

As an attending geneticist, I examined a pediatric patient in my university hospital outpatient genetics clinic who I had diagnosed with a biotinidase deficiency, a rare but treatable inborn error of metabolism. The child presented with intractable seizures but was doing well on daily biotin therapy. The parents informed me that they had never received a bill for my services. They said they would be overjoyed to pay for my services, but they did not know how. I investigated and discovered that our billing department sent invoices to the wrong address. Six months later there was no point in billing their insurance company because it would be "too late" and rejected. The couple ended up making a donation to our research.

Realization: it does not matter how good a physician you are; if you do not bill in a timely fashion you will not get paid.

8. Capital. Commercial laboratories have the ability to purchase state-of-the-art equipment, acquire licenses for genes and technology, and perform clinical validation studies for new assays without having to go through the grant writing, submission, and revision processes that can take months to years before funding is obtained.

Consequently, for high-volume tests, commercial laboratories have slowly but surely accumulated the lion's share of genetic testing to the detriment of academic laboratories.

WHAT ARE THE ADVANTAGES OF ACADEMIC AND REGIONAL LABORATORIES?

Academic and regional laboratories enjoy some advantages over commercial laboratories. Although the most important advantage of commercial laboratories are operational efficiencies, the most important advantage of academic laboratories are clinical information and relationships with patients. The faculties of academic and regional laboratories treat the patients they test. These laboratories have access to clinical information via IT systems and medical records. This allows clinical research to be performed for the development of biomarkers and predictive tests.

Other advantages of academic and regional laboratories include:

1. Early access to new inventions. Inventions developed by the faculty of an institution are immediately available to the laboratory.
2. Access to "free" labor. Principal investigators with salary support from grants, house staff, postdoctoral fellows, graduate students, and medical students are all available to perform research. Training licenses can be obtained so unlicensed individuals can perform clinical testing under supervision of licensed personnel.
3. Less financial pressure. Because publications and grants are still an important currency in academic institutions, the pressure to earn money from testing is somewhat less than in a for-profit, publicly owned corporation.

A MODEST PROPOSAL: THERE IS A PLACE FOR US

Without a paradigm shift, genetic testing will continue to become consolidated into large commercial entities, such as hybrid laboratories and commercial laboratories. A few regional laboratories, including those in large academic medical centers will survive using their own health plan patients and outreach clinics to assure a flow of requisitions. However, the days when every teaching hospital had a cytogenetics, biochemical genetics, and molecular laboratory are nearing an end. I often hear the argument that these laboratories must remain open to teach medical students and house officers, but this may become a luxury that academic medical centers can no longer afford.

Complementary, If Not Complimentary

I believe academic and commercial laboratories can coexist in a mutually beneficial relationship based on cooperation and collaboration rather than competition. Instead of exploiting each other's weaknesses, we can join our strengths to ensure the survival of both commercial and academic laboratories and an optimal climate for genetic testing for patients. The hypothetical, collaborative venture is based on four postulates:

1. Academic laboratories have a vital role to play in translational medicine and the education of medical students, house staff, and postdoctoral fellows.
2. Academic laboratories cannot successfully complete with commercial laboratories for high-volume genetic testing. As discussed above, operational efficiencies, automation, volume purchasing, connectivity, service centers, and insurance company contracts make it impractical for academic laboratories to compete for routine genetic testing.

3. Commercial laboratories have little interest in developing and performing low-volume assays, because these assays are more expensive to run and, owing to CPT coding, may not be better reimbursed by third-party payers.
4. Academic laboratories and commercial laboratories will realize it is in both their interests to collaborate, rather than compete. (This is the toughest one!)

(Euclid required five postulates, so I think I am doing pretty well.)

My proposal is that, rather than competing with each other, academic and commercial laboratories can work together to provide the best possible services for patients and the health care providers who care for them, while also providing appropriate training for medical students, house staff, and fellows.

Education

The educational mission can be shared. Our commercial laboratory accepts residents and fellows for training and the large volumes performed during their rotation assure there is always an interesting and educational series of cases. Trainees who have rotated through our laboratory have found it to be enjoyable and a vital adjunct to their academic experience.

SUMMARY

Academic laboratories could concentrate their efforts in low-volume, highly esoteric assays of interest to their principal investigators and in clinical validation of new biomarkers and assays in the realm of translational medicine. With appropriate collaborative agreements, the academic laboratories could benefit from purchasing concessions, access to patient service centers, sales and marketing forces, and third-party payer relationships. The commercial laboratories could benefit from early access to new and potentially high-volume tests, shared clinical outcome data, and intellectual property.

Large consortia offering a vast menu of routine and esoteric genetic testing under a single umbrella could emerge.[1] This will not be easy. Issues of historical mistrust, animosity, reimbursement, regulation, and funding need to be overcome, but the end result could be fabulous. A brave new world of harmony and service could be ushered in. There is an old adage: one does not make peace with one's friends, only with one's enemies. Perhaps we could then move on to world peace.

REFERENCES

1. Hudson KL, Murphy JA, Javitt GH, et al. Oversight of US genetic testing laboratories. Nat Biotechnol 2006;24:1083–90.
2. Chang JC, Kan YW. A sensitive new prenatal test for sickle-cell anemia. N Engl J Med 1982;307(1):30–2.
3. Strom CM. For the good of the patient: academic and commercial genetic testing laboratories: complementary if not complimentary. Personalized Medicine 2007;4: 489–95.
4. Hofgärtner WT, Tait JF. Characteristics of clinical molecular-genetic testing laboratories in the United States. Clin Chem 1999;45:1288–90.
5. Merz JF, Kriss AG, Leonard DG, et al. Diagnostic testing fails the test. Nature 2002; 415:577–9.
6. Available at: http://oig.hhs.gov/oei/reports/oei-09-00-00200.pdf. Accessed June 19, 2012.

7. Strom CM, Clark DD, Hantash FM, et al. Direct visualization of cystic fibrosis trans-membrane regulator mutations in the clinical laboratory setting. Clin Chem 2004; 50:836–45.
8. Strom CM, Janeszco R, Quan F, et al. Technical validation of a luminex based multiplex assay for 40 mutations in the cystic fibrosis transmembrane regulator protein. J Mol Diagn 2006;8:371–5.
9. Sun W. Nucleic acid extraction and general procedures in molecular diagnostics—techniques and applications for the clinical laboratory. In: Grody W, Nakamura R, Kiechle F, et al, editors. Molecular diagnostics. Amsterdam, Holland: Elsevier Press; 2010. p. 35–58.

Index

Note: Page numbers of article titles are in **boldface** type.

A

Academic pathology departments
  advantages of, 662
  coexisting with commercial laboratories, 662–663
  history of, 653–662
  new business models for, 648–649
  versus commercial laboratories, 660–662
Accreditation Council for Continuing Medical Education, fellowships of, 624
Acquisition, of digital images, 575
Active matrix organic light-emitting diode LCD monitors, 575
Additive color models, 562–563
Alfigen, 656
Alignment, in next-generation sequencing, 591–592
American Board of Pathology, fellowships of, 624
Ampliseq panel, 646
Analytic phase, workflow organization
  anatomic pathology, 612–615
  clinical pathology, 618–619
Anatomic pathology, workflow organization in, 610–617
  analytic phase, 612–615
  cytopathology, 616–617
  laboratory information system role in, 617
  postanalytic phase of, 615–616
  preanalytic phase, 610–612
Assembly, in next-generation sequencing, 591–592
Automation
  disadvantages of, 660
  in clinical pathology, 618–619
  in industrial workflow, 603
Autoverification, of results, 619

B

Banbury Conference, on education programs, 625–628
Barcodes, for workflow, 613, 615
Bayesian Belief Networks-based virtual microscopy model, 630
Bethesda System, for cytopathology, 616
Binary Alignment Map, 595
bioTheranostics, 646
Bit-Map (BMP) files, 566
Broad-Novartis Cancer Cell Line Encyclopedia, 644
Burrow-Wheeler algorithm, for next-generation sequencing, 592

Clin Lab Med 32 (2012) 665–672
http://dx.doi.org/10.1016/S0272-2712(12)00122-9
0272-2712/12/$ – see front matter © 2012 Elsevier Inc. All rights reserved.

labmed.theclinics.com

United States
Postal Service

Statement of Ownership, Management, and Circulation
(All Periodicals Publications Except Requestor Publications)

1. Publication Title	2. Publication Number									3. Filing Date
Clinics in Laboratory Medicine	0	0	0	-	7	1	3			9/14/12

4. Issue Frequency	5. Number of Issues Published Annually	6. Annual Subscription Price
Mar, Jun, Sep, Dec	4	$240.00

7. Complete Mailing Address of Known Office of Publication (Not printer) (Street, city, county, state, and ZIP+4®)	Contact Person
Elsevier Inc. 360 Park Avenue South New York, NY 10010-1710	Stephen R. Bushing Telephone (Include area code) 215-239-3688

8. Complete Mailing Address of Headquarters or General Business Office of Publisher (Not printer)

Elsevier Inc., 360 Park Avenue South, New York, NY 10010-1710

9. Full Names and Complete Mailing Addresses of Publisher, Editor, and Managing Editor (Do not leave blank)

Publisher (Name and complete mailing address)

Kim Murphy, Elsevier, Inc., 1600 John F. Kennedy Blvd. Suite 1800, Philadelphia, PA 19103-2899

Editor (Name and complete mailing address)

Teia Stone, Elsevier, Inc., 1600 John F. Kennedy Blvd. Suite 1800, Philadelphia, PA 19103-2899

Managing Editor (Name and complete mailing address)

Barbara Cohen - Kligerman, Elsevier, Inc., 1600 John F. Kennedy Blvd. Suite 1800, Philadelphia, PA 19103-2899

10. Owner (Do not leave blank. If the publication is owned by a corporation, give the name and address of the corporation immediately followed by the names and addresses of all stockholders owning or holding 1 percent or more of the total amount of stock. If not owned by a corporation, give the names and addresses of the individual owners. If owned by a partnership or other unincorporated firm, give its name and address as well as those of each individual owner. If the publication is published by a nonprofit organization, give its name and address.)

Full Name	Complete Mailing Address
Wholly owned subsidiary of	1600 John F. Kennedy Blvd., Ste. 1800
Reed/Elsevier, US holdings	Philadelphia, PA 19103-2899

11. Known Bondholders, Mortgagees, and Other Security Holders Owning or Holding 1 Percent or More of Total Amount of Bonds, Mortgages, or Other Securities. If none, check box ☐ None

Full Name	Complete Mailing Address
N/A	

12. Tax Status (For completion by nonprofit organizations authorized to mail at nonprofit rates) (Check one)
The purpose, function, and nonprofit status of this organization and the exempt status for federal income tax purposes:
☐ Has Not Changed During Preceding 12 Months
☐ Has Changed During Preceding 12 Months (Publisher must submit explanation of change with this statement)

PS Form 3526, September 2007 (Page 1 of 3 (Instructions Page 3) PSN 7530-01-000-9931 PRIVACY NOTICE: See our Privacy policy in www.usps.com

13. Publication Title		14. Issue Date for Circulation Data Below
Clinics in Laboratory Medicine		September 2012

15. Extent and Nature of Circulation			Average No. Copies Each Issue During Preceding 12 Months	No. Copies of Single Issue Published Nearest to Filing Date
a. Total Number of Copies (Net press run)			407	419
b. Paid Circulation (By Mail and Outside the Mail)	(1)	Mailed Outside-County Paid Subscriptions Stated on PS Form 3541. (Include paid distribution above nominal rate, advertiser's proof copies, and exchange copies)	169	155
	(2)	Mailed In-County Paid Subscriptions Stated on PS Form 3541 (Include paid distribution above nominal rate, advertiser's proof copies, and exchange copies)		
	(3)	Paid Distribution Outside the Mails Including Sales Through Dealers and Carriers, Street Vendors, Counter Sales, and Other Paid Distribution Outside USPS®	76	81
	(4)	Paid Distribution by Other Classes Mailed Through the USPS (e.g. First-Class Mail®)		
c. Total Paid Distribution (Sum of 15b (1), (2), (3), and (4))		▶	245	236
d. Free or Nominal Rate Distribution (By Mail and Outside the Mail)	(1)	Free or Nominal Rate Outside-County Copies Included on PS Form 3541	58	68
	(2)	Free or Nominal Rate In-County Copies Included on PS Form 3541		
	(3)	Free or Nominal Rate Copies Mailed at Other Classes Through the USPS (e.g. First-Class Mail)		
	(4)	Free or Nominal Rate Distribution Outside the Mail (Carriers or other means)		
e. Total Free or Nominal Rate Distribution (Sum of 15d (1), (2), (3) and (4))		▶	58	68
f. Total Distribution (Sum of 15c and 15e)		▶	303	304
g. Copies not Distributed (See instructions to publishers #4 (page #3))		▶	104	115
h. Total (Sum of 15f and g)		▶	407	419
i. Percent Paid (15c divided by 15f times 100)			80.86%	77.63%

16. Publication of Statement of Ownership

If the publication is a general publication, publication of this statement is required. Will be printed
in the **December 2012** issue of this publication.

☐ Publication not required

17. Signature and Title of Editor, Publisher, Business Manager, or Owner		Date
[signature] Stephen R. Bushing – Inventory Distribution Coordinator		September 14, 2012

I certify that all information furnished on this form is true and complete. I understand that anyone who furnishes false or misleading information on this form or who omits material or information requested on the form may be subject to criminal sanctions (including fines and imprisonment) and/or civil sanctions (including civil penalties).

PS Form 3526, September 2007 (Page 2 of 3)

.

Printed and bound by CPI Group (UK) Ltd, Croydon, CR0 4YY

03/10/2024

01040443-0014